ALL IN HER HEAD

MISTY PRATT

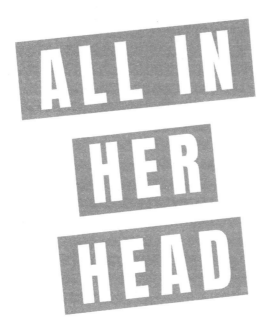

ALL IN HER HEAD

How Gender Bias Harms Women's Mental Health

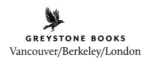

GREYSTONE BOOKS
Vancouver/Berkeley/London

Greystone Books Ltd.
greystonebooks.com

Cataloguing data available from Library and Archives Canada
ISBN 978-1-77840-282-1 (pbk.)
ISBN 978-1-77164-971-1 (cloth)
ISBN 978-1-77164-972-8 (epub)

Editing by Paula Ayer
Copy editing by Crissy Calhoun
Proofreading by Dawn Loewen
Indexing by Stephen Ullstrom
Cover and text design by Belle Wuthrich
Cover illustration from *Sorcellerie, magnétisme, morphinisme, délire des grandeurs*
by Paul Regnard (Paris, 1887), facing page 248

"The Uses of Sorrow" by Mary Oliver
Reprinted by the permission of The Charlotte Sheedy Literary Agency as agent for the author.
Copyright © 2006 by Mary Oliver with permission of Bill Reichblum

Image credits: page 8 courtesy of author; page 24 *Jean-Martin Charcot
Demonstrating Hysteria in a Hypnotised Patient at the Salpêtrière*, etching by
A. Lurat, 1888, after André Brouillet, 1887,
Attribution 4.0, Wellcome Collection; page 205 © Elizabeth Tobin

This book provides general information and discussion about mental health from a
personal, historical, and cultural perspective. It is intended for informational purposes
and does not constitute health or medical advice. The author and the publisher accept no
liability for any damages arising as a result of the direct or indirect application of any
element of the contents of this book.

Printed and bound in the U.K. on FSC® certified paper at CPI Group Ltd. The FSC® label
means that materials used for the product have been responsibly sourced.

Greystone Books thanks the Canada Council for the Arts, the British Columbia Arts
Council, the Province of British Columbia through the Book Publishing Tax Credit,
and the Government of Canada for supporting our publishing activities.

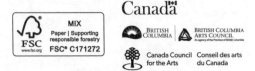

Greystone Books gratefully acknowledges the xʷməθkʷəy̓əm (Musqueam),
Sḵwx̱wú7mesh (Squamish), and səlilwətaɫ (Tsleil-Waututh) peoples on
whose land our Vancouver head office is located.

For Aylen and Emily
That you may always know
the strength and wisdom of your body

CONTENTS

INTRODUCTION

AT SEVENTEEN YEARS OLD, I got sick. The kind of sick that doctors can't diagnose using a blood test or medical technology. The kind of illness that was talked about in whispers, behind closed doors, if it was even talked about at all.

It started on my first morning back to high school after a blissful summer of first love and sun-kissed adventures. It was a bright and warm September day, but when I entered the air-conditioned school, everything suddenly appeared murky and gray. As I stood in the cafeteria, with its waxed floors reflecting the morning sun and students shouting greetings to their friends, a shadow descended over my eyes. Something didn't look right.

I was experiencing a feeling that I couldn't touch or name yet, but which many others have characterized with clichés and worn-out metaphors: the black dog, a rain cloud, a shadow passing across the sun. These are the words and images we use to give life to something that feels like a specter of the self, a distortion of who we truly are. It's also something that seems to exist alone in our minds, growing in strength and power while our bodies grow weaker.

When I look back at this moment, I remember it as the first time I felt the weight of depression. It seemed like the illness came out of nowhere, blocking the sun and transforming my world from color to shades of gray, like the movie *Pleasantville* in reverse. What I later came to understand is that my mental illness wasn't as random as it felt, and that the seeds were sown long before my life fell apart.

Headaches, stomachaches, irritable bowel syndrome, insomnia, panic attacks: all these physical symptoms crept into my life one at a time, but still I did not recognize the darkness for what it truly was. My depression was not "typical" in that my initial blue feelings turned into anxious thoughts and eventually became daily panic attacks. I couldn't get on buses or trains or go into any other place where I felt confined, because my panic revolved around feelings of nausea and a fear of vomiting.

I visited specialists who pressed on my abdomen and stuck a scope down my esophagus, on the hunt for a physical cause of my tummy troubles. All the tests came back negative for any serious illness, and one doctor suggested that I had irritable bowel syndrome. "You need to reduce stress," he said, and I nodded in agreement, unsure of how to do that. My body's internal smoke alarm was beeping, but I couldn't find the source of the fire. I took to popping Zantac, a medication used to reduce stomach acid, every time I felt the familiar stab in my abdomen. Soon it was a daily habit. When I couldn't sleep because of worries over my symptoms, I used Gravol. My weight dropped rapidly, and I began to isolate myself.

Taking a break from school at this point would have been understandable, but it seemed like schoolwork was the only thing tying me to some sense of normality. I was so afraid of failing out of school that the thought of taking time off never crossed my mind.

On an ill-fated family trip, my parents finally realized this was not just "the blues" and wouldn't go away on its own. Back in Canada, they booked the first appointment they could get with our family doctor. My dad did most of the talking, describing my change in mood, sleep, and eating habits. The doctor asked me a few questions about how I was feeling and then heaved a big sigh, shaking his head.

"Why are so many girls dealing with things like this?" he said to no one in particular. This was how I first became aware of the fact that I wasn't alone in my suffering.

HALF OF ALL SERIOUS MENTAL ILLNESS begins in adolescence, but treatment often lags years, or even decades, after diagnosis.[1] Between ages twelve and seventeen, over 36 percent of girls develop depression compared to under 14 percent of boys.[2] And once mental illness begins in adolescence, it often persists throughout a person's adult life, leading to long-term suffering and ongoing mental health care needs.[3]

In teenage land, there are so many moments of vulnerability as we crash through the world with our underdeveloped prefrontal cortex and fluctuating hormones. The brain is scanning the body (for things like heart rate, temperature, and aches and pains), taking input from the senses and past memories, and making second-by-second predictions on what the body needs to survive.[4] How much cortisol should be released to pass our exams, to fit in with the crowd, or to fight for freedom from rules and expectations? What hormonal cocktail will it take to navigate our budding sexuality? And how do we do all of this while toeing the line, fitting ourselves neatly into the confining boxes in which society places us?

The stakes are even higher for girls, when we consider that they are statistically more likely to face sexual violence, harassment, and discrimination.[5] The World Health Organization states that up to one-third of teen girls report their first sexual experience as being "forced."[6] Other research has found that anywhere from 12 to 25 percent of teen girls experience sexual violence at some point before the age of eighteen.[7] Sexual violence, especially if it is repeated or prolonged, may interfere with normal brain development and lead to structural changes in the brain that disrupt psychological well-being well into adulthood.[8]

For many young women, adolescence is the entry point into a mental health system steeped in bias. A long history of treating women's mental and physical illnesses as originating from our baffling female biology (or "weak disposition," as it was later understood) can be traced back to the very first mental disorder attributable to women, described in ancient Greek medicine as "hysteria." Hysteria is where modern psychiatry was born,[9] and I argue that all mental illnesses were first constructed as feminine disorders. This continues to affect the quality of and access to care provided to girls and women.

Mental illness can develop in the perinatal period (defined differently in research, but often referred to as early pregnancy through to one year postpartum) or during menopause, which marks the end of our reproductive years. Over this span of reproductive time and throughout our shifting roles from teen to elder, cisgender women are much more likely to experience mood disorders and anxiety compared with cisgender men, and there is a significant lack of knowledge in general medicine and psychiatry of how our biology and gender roles influence our health and lived experiences.

MY MENTAL ILLNESS STARTED a decade after Prozac, one of the most widely prescribed antidepressants, had hit the market to much fanfare, and medications for mental illness were being aggressively marketed and prescribed to tens of millions of people worldwide.[10] There was a collective sense that mental illness was going to be conquered, and this would be accomplished through the work of biological psychiatry, an approach that treats mental illness as a function of our nervous system. The hypothesis, which is still somewhat influential today, is that depression is caused by lower than normal levels of certain neurotransmitters in the brain, or what's called the "chemical imbalance" theory of mental illness.[11]

As I moved into early adulthood and tried to recover the pieces of my life, I took these medications in the desperate hope that a pill would be the one thing to finally "fix" me. Unfortunately, that wasn't what happened, and I suspect that the difficulties I faced coming off those medications prolonged my suffering. I also spent years in therapy, hopping from one provider to the next, seeking the person who could tell me how to repair what was broken.

My nervous breakdown and search for answers led me through a decades-long exploration of what it means to be "mentally ill" as a girl and woman, the ways in which my symptoms were treated and pathologized, and how unrelenting social pressure and inequality contributed to my ongoing struggles as an unwell woman. Though I was lucky enough to find support through my initial bout of depression and anxiety, I went on to experience repeated relapses throughout my twenties and after the birth of my children. I received multiple mental health diagnoses and spent years in and out of treatments that were expensive and time-consuming. It was not until I became aware of the systemic issues facing girls and women that I was able to find a path toward healing.

In this book, you will read stories shared by other women who have learned to navigate a system in which they are shamed, dismissed, or misdiagnosed. This is not to say that we have not received compassionate care or had positive experiences along the way. There are many care providers who are working hard to change the system, to listen better, and to offer person-centered care. But when we hold a mirror up to our collective experiences, we can see the result of the exhaustion, trauma, and shame that we have experienced individually and as a whole. Only by telling these stories can we fully accept and acknowledge how far we've come and how far we still need to go.

WHEN I SET OUT to write this book, I knew I wanted it to be about women's mental health and mental illness, as it's currently understood by our medical system, culture, and society. As part of my own process, I needed to know why so many women struggle with their mental health, why the current treatment approaches aren't working, and how we could envision a better model for treating women's mental health.

My own journey and the stories shared in this book make it clear that mental wellness is about much more than the psychological side of well-being. Mental health is whole-body health. The pervasive practice of women's physical symptoms and pain being misdiagnosed as mental illness means that women complaining of physical symptoms are often told they're simply stressed out, and their complaints are overlooked or minimized. As I'll show in these pages, women seeking help for their depression and anxiety are facing an arduous journey through a system that is biased toward a capitalist and patriarchal view of health and wellness. Whether it's mental or physical, what ails women seems to always come back to what's in our heads.

The World Health Organization states that less than 2 percent of the global population suffers from severe mental illness such as schizophrenia and bipolar disorders, with rates varying by time period and region but not by gender.[12] These disorders have not increased in prevalence much over time. Where we see a significant rise in mental health problems is in disorders like depression and anxiety, especially among girls and women.[13] Severe mental illness is thought to have a stronger genetic component, whereas mood disorders and anxiety are often attributed to biological risk factors, differences in personality, environment (or culture), and adversity.[14] Within the scope of this book, I focus on what are considered more common mental illnesses, although you'll hear stories from women who have faced similar barriers to treatment for severe mental illness.

I explore the experience of this type of mental distress from a biopsychosocial model,[15] which posits that a combination of biological, psychological, and social factors influence our lived experience. This framework was first proposed in the late 1970s to guide clinicians in their work with patients.[16] As you'll see on the next page in the image I've created based on this model, it suggests that our mental health is influenced by three important factors: our biology (our bodies and brains), our psychology (thoughts, feelings, and emotions), and society (our environment).

In the mid-twentieth century, dissenters within psychiatry advocated to transform the medical model of mental health, which at the time primarily relied on drug treatment.[17] This flavor of psychiatry linked mental disease to a simplistic theory of chemical imbalance of neurotransmitters in the brain, rather than acknowledging that mental illness is likely caused by a complicated mix of social, biological, and psychological causes.

Psychiatrist George Engel called for the integration of psychosocial interventions into mental health care, which he believed would address the multifaceted layers of mental distress. According to Engel, to change how patients were being treated, the entire nature of the discipline of psychiatry needed to shift its focus. Today, many Western practitioners in the field of mental health claim to have adopted a biopsychosocial model of care, but there is not a lot of data to suggest that this is true. Mental illness is still treated largely within the medical model.[18]

Bio-Psycho-Social: A quick reference

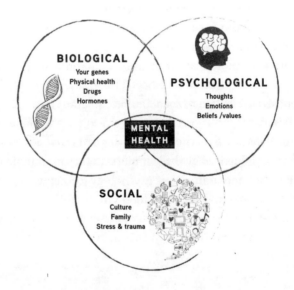

BIOLOGICAL
Your genes
Physical health
Drugs
Hormones

PSYCHOLOGICAL
Thoughts
Emotions
Beliefs /values

MENTAL HEALTH

SOCIAL
Culture
Family
Stress & trauma

The biopsychosocial model is also useful as a lens through which we can understand our own experiences, and how current treatments fail to address the societal pressures we face that contribute disproportionately to women's mental distress.

While I believe that psychiatry and medicine in general have a continuing role to play in the diagnosis and treatment of people struggling with mental illness, there have been limits to what psychiatry has been able to offer me and many others. The treatment model that I navigated as a teen and adult argues that my problems arise from an imbalance in my brain. Yet, as I propose in this book, history reveals that women have continually been slapped with the "unbalanced" label. Whether the culprit is the uterus, ovaries, hormones, or brain chemicals, something about our basic biology is apparently broken. My personal quest for answers became a discovery of my self and a growing understanding that no one treatment could "fix" me. I had never been broken in the first place.

I AM A LOVER OF SCIENCE for all the potential it holds to reveal the solutions for what ails us. The biomedical model of research and health care worships certain types of scientific studies for good reasons: evidence-based medicine needs strong data to support costly medical treatments among so many competing interests. However, the disproportionate focus on data can silence patient experience, increasing the risk that the questions being asked are not the ones that need to be answered.

I'm also aware that historically and presently, men hold the balance of power when it comes to scientific inquiry. Western science has discounted knowledge from women and diverse communities, meaning that what we know about bodies generally refers to white cisgender male bodies. The science that does focus on women's mental health generally includes only cisgender women, which means we are limited when trying to understand the experiences of trans people and gender-diverse people. I use the term "woman" throughout this book to refer to anyone who identifies as a woman (and the term "female" applies to those who were assigned female at birth), although a lot of what I write about could also apply to those who do not identify as women.

This is also a good time to answer a question you might have about this book: "What about men?" Yes, men experience mental illness, too, and yes, they also face barriers in our current system of care. One of the more common explanations I see for men's lower rate of mental illness compared to women's is that women exhibit more "help-seeking" behavior.[19] This means that when women feel bad, they're more likely to visit their doctor and ask for help.[20] However, as I'll address later in this book, this factor alone doesn't explain the difference in mental illness rates between men and women. Furthermore, men's health has been the main attraction in research for a dreadfully long time, while women's health has been largely ignored. We still don't know as much about women's bodies as we do about men's bodies, and I'll review the reasons for this in the first few chapters.

All that aside, I think many men will relate to parts of this book and will perhaps recognize our shared struggles with emotional distress—how women and men are socialized to experience and express emotion differently, and how this influences our ability to seek help as well as our response to treatments.

While I have relied on (mostly Western) scientific evidence in this book, I am equally interested in anecdotal experiences from patients themselves. For too long, women have been told what they think, feel, and experience, and they've even been told that what they think, feel, and experience is all wrong. As we come to better understand our own bodies, and to rely on the inner science of what our bodies are telling us, we can realize this type of knowledge is valid and meaningful. Sharing personal stories also helps us to feel less isolated and can illuminate the hidden systemic forces that are working against all of us.

This book is not prescriptive—I'm not proposing one path to healing that will fit for every woman. All researchers have bias, and I come to the table with lived experience as a white cisgender woman. While I have attempted to highlight the significant additional barriers that women from marginalized groups face in the mental health care system, I do not presume to fully know or understand their lived experiences. I have instead dedicated myself to listening to their stories more fully, acknowledging my immense privilege in this space, and working to eliminate racism and oppression in mental health care.

As a white woman writing about mental health, I also try to avoid falling into the trap of what I call White Woman Wellness Syndrome. Privileged and wealthy white women exhibit symptoms of this syndrome when they assume they know the source of all women's problems and push a simple-fix agenda. Maybe this fix is a culturally appropriative form of Indigenous or religious practices, or maybe it's a trendy diet. Sometimes it's a pile of expensive supplements. Other times women claim "mindset" is the problem, and they tread the dangerous waters of toxic positivity—the belief that we should only cultivate positive thoughts when dealing with serious problems. This syndrome almost always ignores the underlying systemic issues that make it difficult, if not impossible, for some women to access alternative or expensive treatment options. I address those systemic issues because I don't believe we have any hope of making progress on mental health without a firm social strategy.

Finally, when I write about "healing" in this book, I want to make it clear that I'm not talking about being cured—that somehow, we all have the financial and social capacity to magically rid ourselves of mental distress (which places all the responsibility on the individual). Instead, I use "healing" to mean the process I went through to better understand the wider social and cultural factors that affect my own health, and to discover the power (or, sometimes, lack of power) I have to change those factors. On an individual level, I came to know healing as my right to body literacy and bodily autonomy: to know and understand my body, to be in charge of my own medical decisions and outcomes, and to be provided with the same access to proper care and effective treatments as anybody else. Healing is also about shifting our collective understanding of mental well-being; it is not a constant state of joy and happiness, but a deeper knowing that to be human is to be emotional, from the highest of highs to the lowest of lows.

In most chapters, I share personal stories from women I have interviewed for this book, several of whom asked me to change their names to protect their anonymity. I also share my own stories and those of my family. I have interviewed leading experts in neuroscience, psychiatry, psychology, and other disciplines. All these interviews were conducted over Zoom (thank you, pandemic). My work should not be considered an exhaustive exploration of all facets of women's mental health, but I hope it broadens the conversation about what so many of us have faced.

While I have experience in health research, I like to joke that I'm not one of the "ists"—I'm not a psychiatrist, psychologist, neurologist, anthropologist, or sociologist. I have relied on a range of experts and practitioners for clinical expertise, data, and fresh perspectives, but I don't propose that they (or I) have all the answers. Errors in the interpretation of their work are entirely my own. I have settled comfortably in the expert status of someone who has been through the trenches of mental illness, and I hope that my experience, and the experiences of the women who grace these pages, will shed light on the ways in which we can reframe and reclaim women's mental health.

1

HYSTERIA IN ACTION

(In my sleep I dreamed this poem)
Someone I loved once gave me
a box full of darkness.
It took me years to understand
that this, too, was a gift.
MARY OLIVER

I WAS FIVE YEARS OLD the night my grandmother lost her mind. We were winding our way back from the O'Keefe Centre through the dusky streets of Toronto, me with my face plastered to the window of the subway, watching the lines of the tracks disappear underneath the car. Outings with Grandma always promised and delivered—tickets to the ballet or the theater, ice cream treats during intermission, and a ride on the subway—exciting prospects for a girl from the suburbs.

I can't recall if my grandmother seemed distracted or if her behavior pointed to what was to come. My memories of this night are a stack of old photographs that I can flip through at random: a flash of the small postwar home with the old wooden front door and heavy metal knocker; my grandfather sitting in his favorite wingback chair, cold can of beer in hand; and the feelings of fear and confusion that I felt over my grandmother's behavior.

What I don't have is a snapshot of the central player in this story, the one whose mania scaled new heights that night, dropping the bombshell of an extramarital affair (a fabrication, we later determined) and plans for divorce. When we arrived home from the ballet, my grandmother announced she was leaving my grandfather for another man, and a screaming match ensued.

Later, my father would fill in my memories with his own stack of weathered photographs. My mother picking up the phone to hear my grandfather shouting on the other end. My grandmother incoherent and unable to string together a single sentence, which we would later know to be a defining characteristic of her disease. I was called to the phone, told to gather my things, and wait for my father to come pick me up. My clearest memory is standing by the door clutching my suitcase and praying for my father to come.

CHASING THE BALLOON

WHEN WE LOSE OUR MIND, where does it go? Does our identity go along for the ride, drifting off into the ether, or is there a place inside the body where our essence remains? As our mind drifts past, do we jump and try to grab at it, as a young child would chase after a wayward balloon on a windy day? Perhaps we can put up missing-person posters and offer compensation for lost loved ones: *Dorothy Mavis Buckler, born 1923, disappeared on this night in 1985. Reward for her safe return.*

The night my grandma lost her mind was the moment I first became aware of the "mind," described by writer and medical ethicist Harriet A. Washington as "a sort of ghostly extension of the brain into psychic space"[1]—something that is, depending on whom you ask, either fully dependent on the brain or completely separate from the brain. This vague definition means that there is no consensus about where the symptoms of mental illness originate or where they reside. Do they start in the brain and infect the body? Do physical symptoms or physiological causes trigger mental illness? Or does the disease originate in some floating entity called the "mind," something that we can neither quantify nor test in order to make a proper diagnosis?

Wherever it went, my grandmother's mind took regular vacations. In these trips, her world turned shiny and new, filled with possibilities. She was bursting with creative energy, seeking out excitement at every turn. She vacillated between talking a mile a minute and struggling to find her words. For the people responsible for her care, the loss of the mind spelled chaos. Our normal routines were disrupted as my parents and my father's three siblings shouldered the burden of keeping her safe from herself.

Before she got sick, my grandmother was a strongly independent woman living in a world steeped in gender bias and inequality. She began her long career as a teacher in the United Kingdom in a one-room schoolhouse before immigrating to Canada. Later, she became my own school librarian when I attended kindergarten. After her death, I was given a yellowed plastic-bound book with her name typed in faded black lettering on the front page. It was her bachelor's thesis, titled "Positive Roles in Children's Literature," which explored popular children's fairy tales through a feminist lens. I flipped to the introduction and read:

> *Literature is only a small part of most children's environment, and sexism is conveyed in subtle ways. Sex stereotyping pervades our homes, schoolrooms, libraries, television, toys, games, and language. Sex roles are, however, socially conditioned and not innate, and can therefore be changed.*

I sat and read those words over and over, trying to reconcile the grandmother who loomed large in my memories with the woman I would get to know through her writing. She was a woman who completed her bachelor's degree at fifty-nine years old, who taught hundreds of students and instilled in them a love of stories, who chauffeured me around the city to various activities. She was a woman who would blast music on her stereo, joining in with her lovely warbling soprano voice. Never one to shy away from speaking her mind, my grandma was a force to be reckoned with at a time when women and girls were struggling to make themselves seen and heard.

And yet in the privacy of her own home, my grandmother was living with an alcoholic husband who was emotionally abusive to her and his children. Her volatile home life contrasted dramatically with the values she upheld as a woman invested in her career, in the education of children, and in the dismantling of sex stereotyping. I can't help marveling over how she reconciled these two worlds.

DOROTHY (OR KIT, as my grandmother was nicknamed) was an anomaly to the medical community in the early 1980s, because women her age were not normally diagnosed with

bipolar disorder. Once called "manic depression," the disorder (there are several types) leads to dramatic mood swings,
where sufferers can feel on top of the world one week and in
the depths of despair the next. People may also experience
rapid cycling, where moods shift over hours or days, or highs
and lows occur at the same time. But it's generally diagnosed
in a person's teen years or in early adulthood, when changes
in the brain are thought to set off a first episode of mania or
major depression. In recent decades, the study of women's
brains has shown that hormonal triggers in menopause can
also lead to brain changes that give rise to severe mental illness, such as schizophrenia and bipolar disorders.[2] We now
know that older women can develop specific risk factors for
mental health problems, but in the era of my childhood, my
grandmother was seen as an unusual case.[3]

Although the family had been aware of Kit experiencing
some depression in the previous two years, on the night of
our outing and sleepover something in her brain had flipped
the switch to high drive. Her manic episodes were characterized by grandiose ideas, like falling in love with someone
she barely knew, and epic shopping sprees that tallied in the
thousands. She once made a ten-thousand-dollar purchase
of gold jewelry while vacationing in Greece. Other times she
experienced complete breakdowns and lost the ability to
speak. The scariest moment was when she disappeared into
the city, only to be found hours later wandering the streets
confused, not knowing how she'd gotten there.

Mania preceded the inevitable descent into depression,
and it was then that Kit would feel the full weight of her
illness. I remember her physically shrinking, lowering herself into a chair, her shoulders tight and hunched. On visits

to see her at the psychiatric ward, I would sneak a peek at the other residents: young girls, thin as wisps, their wrists wrapped in bandages; middle-aged women wandering the halls, muttering incoherent words to themselves.

Because our family lived only a twenty-minute drive away, the burden of care for my grandmother fell on my parents' shoulders. While lithium seemed to stabilize Kit's ups and downs, her resistance to treatment and her volatile home life with her alcoholic husband meant that she didn't con-sistently take her medication. The smallest shift—a missed dose, an alcoholic drink, a bladder infection—would disrupt the delicate chemistry and trigger another round of drama. Sometimes this would happen while she traveled outside the country, and family members would brace for international rescues when shit hit the fan.

SEARCHING FOR ANSWERS

BEFORE MY GRANDMOTHER received regular psychiatric care, she was in and out of emergency rooms and psychi-atric wards as doctors struggled to understand her symptoms. At the time, there was little cooperation between general medicine and psychiatry, and doctors at first thought Kit was experiencing symptoms of a physical condition rather than a mental health one. My mother also remembers that Kit could be maddeningly lucid during stints in the emergency room, making doctors doubtful that anything was wrong with her mind. When she was asked about alcohol intake, she would confirm she did drink, and doctors assumed that, like her husband, she was an alcoholic. With the lack of research at the time—and still to this day—about mental health in later stages of a woman's life, it's no surprise that medical professionals were baffled by my grandmother's symptoms.

Medical records show that my grandmother was prescribed four different medications: an anticonvulsant, an antipsychotic, a benzodiazepine, and an antidepressant (which was stopped after it led to further manic episodes). Her physical symptoms confused doctors, as they mimicked a transient ischemic attack (a ministroke)—loss of speech or garbled speech, delirium, and tremors. Doctors mulled over multiple diagnoses before settling on bipolar.

There has always been an inkling of doubt in my mind as to what my grandmother was truly grappling with—whether her physical symptoms were indicative of a disease that involved both the mind and the body. I am positive that mental health problems played a role in her symptoms, but I sometimes wonder if a more nuanced understanding of whole-body health may have led to a more positive outcome for Kit.

As we'll discuss in Chapter 5, mental health diagnoses are determined by a doctor's clinical profile of a patient, which is highly subjective and prone to bias. Two illnesses that have overlapping symptoms with bipolar are borderline personality disorder (BPD)[4] and conversion disorder.[5] Both are modern interpretations of hysteria—a diagnosis women used to receive when they experienced dissociative symptoms (feelings of detachment from oneself or reality), which were often related to trauma. Women continue to receive these diagnostic labels at much higher rates than men, and they face long and confusing paths toward an eventual diagnosis that fits—often racking up a dizzying mix of physical and mental diagnoses on the way.

When she wasn't hospitalized, Kit occasionally stayed with us until it was safe for her to return home. This became more important after my grandfather passed away and she was living alone. Her illness eventually necessitated a forced move to a nursing home, where she lived out the last twenty years of her life. She loudly opposed this decision and never fully accepted that she had a mental illness.

Several years ago, I sat down with a box of family files stored at my parents' house. As I pored over handwritten and typed letters, newspaper clippings, and black-and-white photographs, I learned that the curse of mental illness had touched the lives of at least two other women in my family tree, both following childbirth. In my grandfather's hastily transcribed memoirs, I read that my paternal great-grandmother stayed in a "nursing home" after the birth of her third child. Even more tragic was the story of my grandmother's sister, who died by suicide shortly after the birth of twins.

As a young child, I had heard some of these stories but understood none of the underlying meaning. Our family history was laid out like facts scribbled onto a chalkboard, but the deeper context of what "mental illness" meant was something I did not have the tools to explore. What I came to observe was that emotions were as uncontrollable and fickle as the changing weather. Pure joy was a form of madness, and despair was a pit into which you could fall forever. I see now that I strived to settle myself in the middle, to push back on emotions that I didn't want to feel.

It wasn't until I was seventeen, when I found myself in the office of a child psychologist in the throes of my mental breakdown, that I would be forced to face my own box full of darkness. For many years, I believed this box would contain answers: the reasons for my breakdown and a clear picture of the genetic imprints I carried. But mental illness has no single cause, and many scientists no longer believe our genes play a starring role.[6] Emotions and mental problems are complex, just as our brains are complex organs, predicting our bodies' needs at any given moment.

Our social world may play a much bigger role than we think, especially when it comes to how women's "problems of the mind" are diagnosed and treated. The echoes of the myth of female hysteria can still be heard today, but it is in the past where our story begins.

A (VERY) SHORT HISTORY OF HYSTERIA

NEITHER OF MY PARENTS RECALL whether my grandmother received a diagnosis of hysteria, but what is apparent in her narrative is that (at least in the early stages of her illness) most clinicians acted as though her symptoms were exaggerated or arose from emotional distress, despite the range of physical symptoms she was also experiencing. She was often sent home without any support, and seeing a new psychiatrist each time she visited the emergency department meant that there was no coordinated care.

In 1980, the year I was born and around the time my grandmother started experiencing symptoms of bipolar, the third edition of the *Diagnostic and Statistical Manual of Mental Disorders* (DSM) removed hysteria (a term derived from the Greek word for uterus) from its growing list of mental health disorders. However, a diagnosis of a different name popped up in its place: conversion disorder—a term coined by the founder of psychoanalysis, Sigmund Freud. It has also been called functional neurologic disorder, and the U.S. National Institutes of Health now lists the condition under "Genetic and Rare Diseases."[7] The word "conversion" refers to an individual's somatic (or bodily) symptoms that Freud claimed were due to repressed conflict or trauma; he argued that these repressed emotions converted into physical symptoms.[8]

In conversion disorder, individuals are experiencing serious physical symptoms that cannot be explained by a medical condition. These might include neurological symptoms such as trouble walking, numbness, involuntary movement (such as tics), or even seizures. When modern medicine can find no cause, patients are relegated to a catchall diagnosis that could more honestly be labeled "We're not entirely sure what is wrong with you." Historically, medicine has diagnosed physical ailments not yet fully understood—advanced syphilis being one example[9]—as psychological conditions, and this trend continues today.[10] In my grandmother's case, doctors seemed to skip over her physical symptoms to diagnose a mental illness. In a modern system that claims to understand that there is no strict dividing line between the mental and the physical, women continue to be on the receiving end of stereotypical mental diagnoses that further stigmatize their distress.

Before conversion disorder became the diagnosis du jour, hysteria dominated in the late nineteenth and early twentieth centuries' burgeoning field of mental health. In their book *How the Brain Lost Its Mind: Sex, Hysteria, and the Riddle of Mental Illness*, Allan H. Ropper, a neurologist and professor of neurology at Harvard Medical School, and mathematician Brian David Burrell write that symptoms of this disorder could "run the gamut from migraine to paralysis, numbness, fainting, sweats, difficulty in breathing, insomnia, and even nymphomania."[11] It was French neurologist Jean-Martin Charcot who took the mystery of hysteria to the "stage" by parading afflicted women in clinical lessons at the Salpêtrière Hospital in the late nineteenth century. In André Brouillet's well-known painting *A Clinical Lesson at the Salpêtrière*, Charcot is pictured lecturing to a group of eager male practitioners who are observing a patient (Marie "Blanche" Wittmann) in the throes of hysteria.[12] Her hand is bent at the wrist and tightly held in a fist, and she seems to either have fainted or be in a state of hypnosis, which Charcot believed could cure hysteria. One wonders if her state of partial undress is what's holding the attention of the men in the room.

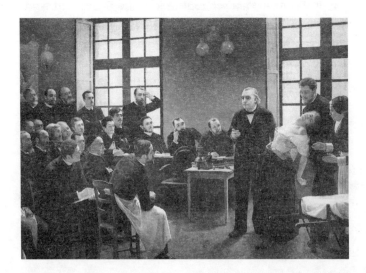

Interestingly, Charcot argued against the gendered prejudice of the disease; he taught that hysteria had organic (biological) causes and could affect both men and women. Despite his claim, for much of the nineteenth and twentieth centuries, hysteria was a label primarily applied to women. This is still the case today, with more women being diagnosed with conversion disorder than men.[13] It was believed men couldn't suffer from hysteria because of their lack of a uterus—or, more precisely, a "wandering uterus," because that's what ancient Greek society believed was the cause of such distressing symptoms. The wandering womb had the potential to place pressure on a number of organs, which could lead to both physical and mental symptoms. Hysteria was born as an illness with a physical cause.

Over the centuries, the notion of hysteria weaseled its way outside the confines of the medical system and became embedded in religion, culture, and broader civilization. Mark Micale writes in *Approaching Hysteria: Disease and Its Interpretations* that the origins of the medical concept of hysteria shifted (from around the fifth to the thirteenth century) into "a manifestation of innate evil"—in other words, hysterical women were thought to be possessed by the devil rather than suffering a physical malady.[18] This brought about different treatments that were less medical and more supernatural, like prayers, charms, incantations, and exorcisms.

By the Middle Ages, the idea that hysteria was caused by the wily uterus had been largely abandoned; medieval European society shifted its focus from hysteria as a medical diagnosis to a wider discourse about women as demonic, sinful, and contaminated.[14] Led by both the Catholic and Protestant churches, the witch hunts from the late fifteenth century until the late eighteenth century in Europe tried approximately eighty thousand "witches" and executed around half of them.[15] (While some of them were men, the vast majority of witches were women.)

Some writers, like Sander Gilman and colleagues in *Hysteria Beyond Freud*, document the various explanations for the rise of the notion of witchcraft, proposed as men's invention intended to silence women's discourse "with the animals and plants, the trees and birds, even the clouds and the moon," or as a way to suppress female sexuality.[16] There is also the argument in Barbara Ehrenreich and Deirdre English's book *Witches, Midwives, and Nurses* that the earliest accusations of witchcraft in Europe grew from the fear of female healers competing with church-affiliated male doctors.[17]

Official manuals for the detection of witches came with instructions for the torture and execution of women who committed any among a range of crimes: blasphemy, religious heresy, lewdness, and, in Ehrenreich and English's words, "every conceivable sexual crime against men. Quite simply, they [were] 'accused' of female sexuality."[19]

As the smoke settled around the burning stakes of the seventeenth-century witch hunts, hysteria as a biological problem rose again from the ashes. It was the physician Edward Jorden and his contemporaries who argued that women's diseases were medical problems to be cured and not demons that needed to be exorcised.[20] His book, published in 1603 and titled *A Briefe Discourse of a Disease Called the Suffocation of the Mother*, revived the wandering womb concept, arguing that the roving uterus could cause "suffocation" by placing pressure on other organs.[21] (The word "mother" in the title refers to the uterus.) He claimed (completely seriously) that this led to "suffocation in the throate, croaking of Frogges, hissing of Snakes... frenzies, convulsions, hickcockes, laughing, singing, weeping, crying." The cure for womb suffocation was a prescription of fasting, sleeping, and praying. A woman who paid strict attention to this diet of deprivation, and who could control her thoughts, emotions, and desires, would ultimately be cured.[22]

In the eighteenth century, there were changing and competing theories about the nature of hysteria. Women's nervous afflictions were often labeled hysteria by medical professionals but were also sometimes called vapors, spleen, or melancholy.[23] The disease was increasingly lumped into a set of various nervous disorders and diagnosed in both men and women, but as might be expected, it was much more common among women (especially white women in the upper classes of society). Violent treatments were proposed to tackle the most extreme cases, including excessive bloodletting, leeching, induced vomiting, and laxatives, all designed to silence and punish female patients in the ultimate goal of maintaining strict gender roles.[24]

THIS BRINGS US BACK to the late nineteenth century, and what I imagine to be hysteria's penultimate heyday (with Freud making the final, and perhaps most effective, effort to reinvent the concept). Toward the end of Charcot's life, and under pressure from much of the research community, he backed down from his hypothesis of hysteria as a physical disease and conceded it was mainly psychological in nature.[25] This matched the dominant wave of thought that had arisen in the early medical communities of the seventeenth century, which insisted that mental disorders were solely located in the mind, and physical disorders were located by some measurable means in the body. The medical community could then wrest the body from the control of the church (which saw body and soul as one divine being and prohibited study of the body through dissection), thus paving the way for scientific inquiry and medical study.[26]

Freud's theory was that hysteria's physical symptoms stemmed from unconscious motivations, such as trauma from sexual abuse. Or to put it another (weirder) way, "this psychological damage was a result of removing male sexuality from females, an idea that stems from Freud's famous 'Oedipal moment of recognition' in which a young female realizes she has no penis, and has been castrated," as Ada McVean recounts for McGill University's Office for Science and Society.[27] Freud's belief that hysteria arose because women were sad over the loss of their male genitalia forever linked the female psyche to the disease, driving the next seventy-five years or so of psychiatric care. Hysteria moved out of our uterus and ovaries and headed straight for our minds.

It would be easy to point the finger at both Charcot and Freud as the top influencers in our modern understanding of hysteria, now known as conversion disorder, and the ones directly responsible for the reclassification of traditionally "hysterical" symptoms as anxiety, obsessive-compulsive disorders, manic depression, and borderline personality disorder. However, these two individuals followed and preceded a long line of elite scientists and doctors—all men—who built a very powerful belief system that positioned the female body and mind as deficient.

For instance, Charles Darwin gave us the theory of evolution, but he also argued that evolution made males superior to females. In *The Descent of Man, and Selection in Relation to Sex*, he proposes that the "chief distinction in the intellectual powers of the two sexes is shewn by man attaining to a higher eminence, in whatever he takes up, than woman can attain—whether requiring deep thought, reason, or imagination, or merely the use of the senses and hands." Thus, he concludes, "man has ultimately become superior to woman."[28] In her book *Inferior*, science journalist Angela Saini details personal correspondence from an early women's rights activist, Caroline Kennard, to Darwin, in which she asks him to clarify this statement. In his reply, Darwin doubles down on his theory, telling Kennard that "I certainly think that women though generally superior to men [in] moral qualities are inferior intellectually."[29]

While we can't ignore or dismiss the historical importance of the work of scientists like Darwin, it's vital that we continue to challenge the enduring legacy of male-supremacist theories if we hope to address the sexism women face in our twenty-first-century mental health care system.

I'VE STUDIED THE IDEA of hysteria across the ages and have found that the concept has a dizzying array of interpretations at any given time. Mark Micale concludes in his book that hysteria has been situated in "the womb, the abdomen, the nerves, the ovaries, the mind, the brain, the psyche, and the soul. [Hysteria] has been construed as a physical disease, a mental disorder, a spiritual malady, a behavioral maladjustment, a sociological communication, and as no illness at all."[30] If the concept of hysteria is so pervasive across centuries, across our bodies, across our language and discourse on femininity, it's not a stretch to suggest that hysteria has permeated our modern world in similar ways, specifically as mental disorders that are disproportionately diagnosed in women.

It's highly unlikely that care providers in today's medical system believe nonsense about wandering wombs, weak nerves, or our supposed unconscious desire for a penis. However, the enduring effects of the hysteria label mean that women are often treated as if they're wanting in some way— wanting in character, strength, courage, or gumption to pick themselves up by the bootstraps and get on with things. The gendered language we use to talk about mental health also paints a picture of women who are "overly emotional," "hormonal," or "crazy." We are not enough and we are too much, somehow all at the same time. The history of hysteria and the ways it continues to bleed through to our modern health care system mean that women are being diagnosed and medicated for having emotions that we share with all humans, but which society sees as abnormal or undesirable when they're exhibited by a woman.

2

GENDER BIAS IN MENTAL HEALTH CARE

The solution to the sex and gender data gap is clear: We have to close the female representation gap. When women are involved in decision-making, research, in knowledge production, women do not get forgotten.

CAROLINE CRIADO PEREZ[1]

RECENTLY, MY DAUGHTER was given a wooden jigsaw puzzle for her birthday. It came with six small pieces that slotted together to form a three-dimensional star. It took four adults and two children several hours to figure out the puzzle, because each piece needed to be perfectly placed to snap the star together.

This puzzle is a lot like women's mental health: it can be tricky (and often frustrating) to piece together. There is strong data to suggest that women experience depression and anxiety at much higher rates than men, but *why* this is the case is still up for debate. First, let's take apart the issue piece by piece—beginning with the linchpin: our medical system.

THE MALE BODY AS DEFAULT

TO THIS DAY, models of health and disease treat the male body as the default human body, thanks (once again) to our good friends the ancient Greeks, who had a whole host of wacky ideas about the deficiencies of the female body.[2] If we go back to the beginning (in Biblical terms, but after the ancient Greeks), early Christian theology interpreted Eve as inferior to Adam, given that God made her by taking his rib. Within this narrative of human creation, not only are female bodies a kind of afterthought, but we required a helping hand from a male body simply to come into existence. And while creationism isn't a belief that the majority of people hold in the U.S., a 2019 Gallup poll showed that 40 percent of American adults continue to believe that the story of Genesis reflects how man and woman were created not as equals but as opposites: leader/follower, dominant/subordinate, and active/passive.[3]

Modern medicine has come far from Aristotle's belief that the female body was a deformed male body,[4] but the female body remains shrouded in mystery: not because our biology is fundamentally mysterious, but because medical literature on female health and disease is either lacking or nonexistent.

One factor contributing to this gap is the lack of women's representation at the top of the educational system. Women in medical professions continue to be underrepresented in senior faculty or leadership roles, and they often face more barriers in building successful research careers.[5] There are also fewer women leading clinical research institutes and research teams.

Physicians go through a long process to become educated and certified; they are taught, trained, and mentored throughout their education and careers within a patriarchal medical model. If women are not able to hold positions of power within the medical system, there are trickle-down effects as to which clinical issues receive funding, which diseases are researched, and which topics are taught in medical schools.

There is also a long and storied history of women being marginally represented in or outright banned from medical research trials.[6] One big reason for this was the tragedy of thalidomide—a sedative that was prescribed to thousands of pregnant women in the late 1950s and early 1960s to help with morning sickness and which resulted in babies being born with severe limb deformities. As the medical community grappled with this grave error, the Food and Drug Administration published a 1977 guidance document that advised researchers to exclude women of "childbearing potential" from clinical trial research.[7] The risk to such a vulnerable population was thought to be too great.

A sweeping ban meant that almost all women were excluded from trial participation, even if they were extremely unlikely (and didn't desire) to become pregnant. The guidance also took away the opportunity for women and researchers to use their own judgment to assess risk. Given the choice, some women would have opted to participate in studies based on their personal assessment of the risks and benefits.

It wasn't just thalidomide that kept women out of clinical trials. There was an unfounded belief in the scientific world that female data was "messier," or prone to being skewed because of fluctuating hormones, which necessitated exclusion from all stages of research: laboratory studies using human cells, animal studies, and clinical trials in humans. The ironic truth that's since been uncovered is that men are actually "more hormonal," if you consider day-to-day fluctuations compared to fluctuations over the entire menstrual cycle.[8]

In 1993, U.S. Congress passed a law that required women and minorities to be included in all clinical research and stated that trials needed to be designed to analyze whether the drugs (or other interventions) being studied affected women and underrepresented populations differently.[9] Other countries went on to publish policy documents and guidelines, but efforts have been fragmented and researchers argue that this has stalled progress.

In the last decade, funding agencies around the world have released guidance and stipulations for incorporating sex- and gender-based variables into health care research. The U.S. National Institutes of Health mandated the inclusion of sex as a biological variable in 2016, followed by the Canadian Institutes of Health Research in 2019.[10] In 2021, the European Commission's Horizon Europe program reaffirmed its commitment to gender equality in research and now requires researchers to integrate gender as a separate variable.[11]

SEX OR GENDER: YOU CAN'T STUDY ONE WITHOUT THE OTHER

THE GOOD NEWS is efforts to level the field in medical research seem to be making a difference. Researchers are directed (sometimes by law and sometimes by their funders) to include females in studies and to show how they're analyzing data by sex. The bad news is we still have a lot of confusion around what "sex" and "gender" mean for research and health.

First, a couple of basic definitions, because I'm using the terms "female" and "woman" interchangeably in this chapter, and that can muddle things. In biology, our sex is multi-dimensional, involving genes, our anatomy (genitals, uterus, ovaries), and hormones.[12] Gender is defined as the norms, behaviors, and roles typically associated with being a woman or a man, which can vary from society to society and change over time as well as expand beyond binary identities.[13]

Over centuries, medical knowledge separated the biological male and female into distinct categories, with females as the inferior members of the species. But recent discoveries have proposed that the two sexes are not so dissimilar after all. As zoologist Lucy Cooke says in *The Guardian*, "The things that drive you down the male or female pathway are basically the same genes, just playing a different tune,"[14] which means that the boundary between the sexes is not as rigid as we once thought. Variations in sex characteristics and behaviors have been observed all over the animal kingdom, raising the question: If it's messier than we once thought, how do we, as Cooke says, "embrace the chaos"?

In a traditionally patriarchal view, female sex characteristics have been closely linked to the state of our physical and mental health, and the myth that our anatomy can cause illness and disease is as old as ancient Greece. Stereotypically, our sex is also married to our emotional state; females are viewed as much more likely to experience mental distress due to our biology. When it comes to gender, the hormonally unbalanced or unstable woman is a culturally constructed idea. Both men and women feed into this narrative when we speak of "raging hormones" and mood swings. Simply stating "I'm on my period" is code for "This is why I'm behaving in this way."

Putting stereotypes aside, sex differences in mood and anxiety disorders have been discovered in research comparing males with females, yet few studies are paying attention to gender *and* sex factors that may make both females (as a biological category) and women (as a social category) more vulnerable to mental health issues.[15] The scientific establishment often muddles the differences between sex and gender, linking our biology to harmful gendered stereotypes about women. As Elinor Cleghorn writes in *Unwell Women: Misdiagnosis and Myth in a Manmade World*, "not all women have uteruses and not all people who have uteruses, or who menstruate, are women," but medicine and research have traditionally treated "woman" and "female" as one and the same.[16]

The very question of "what makes us different" can obscure knowledge about how sex and gender influence each other.[17] For example, are men more muscular because of the sex hormone testosterone, or have they learned gendered behaviors (such as working out at the gym to build more muscle) that have changed how testosterone is expressed in their bodies? When we treat sex or gender as a strict binary, we also risk excluding people who have differences in sexual development (they don't fall neatly into male or female categories) or who don't identify as either a man or woman.

To gain further clarity in how sex and gender are studied in health research, I reached out to Liisa Galea, a world-renowned researcher, senior scientist, and Treliving Family Chair in Women's Mental Health at the Centre for Addiction and Mental Health, who explores how sex and stress hormones affect the brain and mental health across the life span.

"The thing that I try to say is don't be afraid of sex differences. I think people are afraid because it somehow means that one sex is lesser than the other—that's not what the research shows in any way, shape, or form," says Galea. "It shows the process is very different in one sex versus the other sex. And if we ignore that, which is what the literature has done, it costs us lives."

Galea has largely focused on the absence of sex-specific data in health research, and you'll hear more from her about this in the next chapter. In a study investigating both human and animal studies published in six neuroscience and psychiatry journals from 2009 to 2019, Galea and coauthors found that only 5 percent of studies in 2019 (up from 2 percent in 2009) used an appropriate analysis for the discovery of possible sex differences in the outcomes.[18] "There are plenty of studies that use both males and females, men and women, and gender-diverse individuals, but they don't analyze by it," says Galea, which means that statistical methods can't reveal how sex might impact a female's (or male's) response to a treatment.

Galea underscores that we also need to consider individual factors such as age, race, and socioeconomic status, or we risk comparing females as a homogeneous group to the dominant male body. What we really need are more studies comparing females to females, to reveal individual (and gendered) factors that will help us determine what solutions might work best for each person. I identify as a woman and was assigned female at birth, but I am not the same woman or female that you might be. We may overlap quite a bit, but we can also differ by age, race, body type, sexual orientation, socioeconomic status, and ability (among many other factors).

Let's explore a case study for why we need better clarity and more nuance in sex- and gender-based research. The sedative drug zolpidem, which you may know as Ambien, was first approved by the U.S. Food and Drug Administration (FDA) for the treatment of insomnia in 1992. Once it was on the market, reports began circulating that women were experiencing side effects of next-day drowsiness and driving impairment. After decades of these reports, the FDA recommended giving women lower doses than men.

But plot twist: though findings did reveal sex-specific differences in drug clearance (the rate at which the body eliminates the drug), further research didn't find any differences in drowsiness or driving impairment, meaning the FDA got it wrong.[19] The researchers who dove deep into the science of zolpidem concluded that dosage reduction recommendations have led to *underdosing* in some women, which would inadequately treat insomnia. The research also found individual variations in response to the drug (meaning some people could experience longer bouts of drowsiness than others), underscoring the need to explore differences *between* females.[20]

Zolpidem is a clear case for how sex and gender interactions matter. For a woman experiencing insomnia, there are likely multiple intersectional factors impacting her sleep. Is she a mother who wakes multiple times in the night to tend to her children? Is she experiencing financial stress that can interfere with good nutrition and sleep? Is she working night shifts? Unanswered questions remain, but one thing is apparent: just studying sex differences without considering other factors is not going to help us in our quest for improved mental health research.

I ASK GALEA what's more important—biology or sociology—when it comes to brain health and mental illness, and she tells me I'm asking the wrong person. "I'm going to say biology is number one," she says. But she adds a caveat: "We already know it's genes by environment." What she means is that the expression of genes is influenced by our environment, which includes our external world (our culture, social support, adversity we face, environmental chemicals) and our internal world (our hormones and metabolism, for instance). "I don't think you can pit one against the other," she says. "You can't remove the biology, so that's why we can't remove sex. And you can't remove the environment, so don't remove the gender." Sex matters *and* gender matters, so it's time for researchers to analyze both.

At the risk of oversimplifying sex and gender in my own telling of this story, let's look at the gender gap in mental health. We'll come back to biology and mental health in the next chapter, but keep in mind that sex and gender overlap in many ways, and I will sometimes refer to both together.

THE GENDER GAP IN PREVALENCE, DIAGNOSIS, AND TREATMENT

DESPITE (OR PERHAPS BECAUSE OF) a growing awareness of the importance of mental health and a much wider acceptance of people seeking treatment for their problems, rates of more common mental illnesses have significantly increased over the past several decades. While rates of severe mental illness have remained steady over time and don't differ much by gender, there are gender differences in the rates of more common mental disorders, including depression and anxiety. Prevalence rates vary across cultures, but throughout the world, data has shown that women are approximately twice as likely as men to be diagnosed with depression.[21]

Though many will point the finger at the COVID-19 pandemic, which was widely reported to have caused a big surge in people reporting symptoms of anxiety and depression, a 2023 systematic review found otherwise—*except* for women. Even then, they found only a slight deterioration in the mental health of women/females compared to men/males, although it's good to keep in mind that this data was all survey-based.[22] Examining health data such as medical records may provide more accuracy, although it wouldn't capture people seeking care from private providers or those who don't seek care at all.

As I write this three years after the start of the pandemic, survey data continues to emerge that shows mental health problems and substance use remain elevated.[23] Time will tell if these trends represent an accurate picture of what the mental health system sees on the ground (in terms of treatment and service use), but a consistent finding in data before and during the pandemic is that anxiety and depression symptoms are more pronounced for women.

Why is that?

In a 2017 study in *The Lancet Psychiatry*, Christine Kuehner identifies several possible causes for the gender gap in depression, including:

- Biological variables, such as genes and sex hormones (although she notes that evidence for this explanation is scarce);

- Women's diminished stress response (we are more likely to release less cortisol during stressful events, which is associated with a higher risk of subsequent depression even after the event has passed);

- Individual factors, like lower self-esteem and higher risk for rumination and body-related shame;

- Higher rates of traumatic childhood experiences (such as physical and sexual abuse); and

- Lack of gender equality, lower access to resources, and lower social status spheres.[24]

When it comes to diagnosis, women are often assessed differently than men. One of the examples Liisa Galea gives me is in the diagnosis of major depressive disorder (MDD). "For something like MDD, females have 'atypical' symptoms," she says. "Women are more likely to show anxiety, and that's considered 'atypical' depression. Is it really atypical? Or has it been that, historically, men and males have been studied, and so therefore the expression of depression in them is what's held up as the standard?"

Even though the majority of people presenting with depression are women, somehow we're considered the odd ones out. Galea says that this means "the disease risk, the manifestation of the disease, and the treatment of disease can be very sex specific." What's likely to work as a treatment for most men may not work for most women. And when women are clinically screened for a mood disorder, a care provider may miss a diagnosis of depression if the woman reports that anxiety is her dominant symptom.

Gender and sex differences have also been documented in responses to mental health medications and in adverse reactions.[25] When women are included in clinical trials, variables such as hormonal contraceptives, menstrual cycles (which mean differing responses to medication at different points in our cycles), pregnancy, childbirth, and menopause have been found to affect treatment outcomes. These variables sometimes lead researchers to exclude women from participating in research altogether.[26] The pandemic gave us a good example of how medical research disregards women's health: many individuals tried to report menstrual cycle changes following COVID-19 vaccination, and at first these claims were dismissed.[27] Thankfully, after much media coverage and female researchers pushing for the data to be tracked, a large study validated these reports. They found that there was a temporary change in menstrual cycle length but no change in the number of days people bled.[28] "We have immune signals in our endometrium... so of course, there's going to be an immune response," says Galea.

Even when sex or gender is considered in research, things can be different in frontline care. Social and psychological factors particular to women, like the ones identified in the *Lancet Psychiatry* paper, are often ignored. A woman presenting to a doctor with mental health symptoms may be experiencing physical or sexual violence in the home, conflict at work, or grief after the death of a loved one. Rather than the doctor building a treatment plan that's appropriate to her needs and the resources available to her, the patient embarks on a circuitous journey through the mental health care system that comes with significant individual, social, and economic costs. For other women, caregiving burdens can be a barrier to participation in treatments that would help them to recover. Trying to find care for a young child or elderly parent in order to attend a one-hour therapy appointment can be a big challenge.

ALL THINGS BEING EQUAL, a man and a woman who each seek medical care for similar symptoms should receive the same assessment and similar diagnosis, with a treatment plan that takes personal factors into account. But this isn't what happens. Even with identical lists of diagnostic criteria in front of them, and even when the patients are exhibiting similar symptoms, doctors are more likely to diagnose a woman than a man with a mental disorder. In a 2020 study of over eight thousand individuals in Spain, women were almost 2.5 times as likely as men to be diagnosed with anxiety and depression, even after controlling for mental health status (which means the researchers wouldn't overestimate this difference if women's distress was truly worse).[29]

Our foray into hysteria and gender bias has shown us how the insidious belief that women's bodies are responsible for our moods leads many in the medical community (and even women themselves) to see these moods as requiring medical treatment.[30] At the same time, the gender-based risk factors we have explored (which intertwine with biological risk factors) may lead women to use the medical system more than men, often to address concerns with depression or anxiety. One theory is that dominant forms of masculinity in many cultures discourage men from expressing feelings of depression or anxiety, which could mean that men are being underdiagnosed.[31]

In the Spanish study I referenced above, the researchers discovered a significant gender gap *despite* controlling for women's higher rates of health care visits. They make two important points worth mentioning here:

1. The "social causality" perspective on poor mental health can help to explain how gender-based discrimination, violence, and inequality lead to higher rates of anxiety and depression in women (more to come on this in Chapter 6).

2. We need to equally consider "social labeling," which is when normal experiences are medicalized, leading to overdiagnosis of mental health issues, particularly for women.[32]

ARE WOMEN REALLY MOODIER THAN MEN?

THE IDEA OF SOCIAL LABELING brings up an important question: Are women labeled as more emotional and therefore more prone to mental illness?

First, a short primer on the psychology of mood and emotion. Emotions are thought to be fleeting, and the consensus in cognitive and psychological research is that they depend on a trigger, or a "stimulus."[33] Your partner makes a snide remark about the kitchen being messy, anger wells up in you, and you snap back, "Well, *clean it* then!" Or you watch *Moana* with your kids and find yourself sniffling into a tissue when Moana's grandmother comes back as a spirit stingray (true story).

A mood state is generally thought to be longer lasting than an emotion. You might say something like, "I'm in a great mood today!" when you tick off all the boxes on your to-do list, spend quality time with your children and partner, and manage to fit in that elusive "me time." Alternately, a bad-mood kind of day might be when you wrap yourself in a blanket burrito and spoon ice cream from a bucket while you binge-watch *The Crown*.

The temporary emotions and short-term moods we feel and express can lead to longer mood states such as depression or anxiety. These diagnoses are made when symptoms occur over a period of time (generally two weeks), but it is important to understand that the basis of mood states is our fleeting and dynamic emotions.[34]

Research has framed emotion as a stimulus-response process in the brain that happens when we react to something around us. This traditional understanding identifies five basic emotions—happiness, sadness, anger, fear, and disgust—which we express in stereotypical ways.[35] These relate to how our body language and facial expressions display an emotion—are we scrunching up our nose, dropping our jaw, making an O shape with our mouth, smiling, or grimacing? The common consensus, up until the past decade, was that humans all over the world share these same emotions, and there are universal and distinct patterns of brain processes involved in our body-based feeling and emotional expression. One neuroscientist, whom you'll meet in the next pages, has challenged traditional emotion theory and made waves in the field of cognitive science.

Stereotypes about emotions have also been gendered, rooted in a pervasive sociocultural belief that women are more emotional than men. When asked to describe their feelings from memory, females report feeling more frequent momentary emotion than males, on average.[36] However, when those same people recorded their emotional experiences over a day, there were no sex differences. Despite this evidence, Western society does an excellent job of perpetuating gender-based stereotypes when it comes to emotions. Take, for example, an arguing heterosexual couple. We see a multitude of examples in movies and TV shows where the man gets angry and punches a hole in the wall and the woman runs from the room, sobbing into her hands. Women cry, while men get angry and physically violent. These depictions feed the narrative and reinforce that men should only express themselves in angry and powerful ways, even though the reality is that men experience fear and sadness just as much as women do.

If we look at brain structure, there is no strong evidence of any structural sex differences that lead to functional differences—meaning we can't show that sex differences in brain structure lead females to behave differently than males. As Lisa Feldman Barrett, a leading researcher in the field of psychology and neuroscience, puts it: "When scientists extrapolate from small differences to 'his brain, her brain,' they are practicing essentialism. This is because the differences—which are summaries across groups of individuals who vary from one another (not all women are alike, not all men are alike) and whose distributions overlap—are assumed to be present in every single male and female brain and invariant in time and place, due to some fixed, genetic blueprint."[37] We can't take what we learn from a small sample of brain imaging and conclude that this is true across all males and all females.

There is also important work to be done to explore differences within the heterogeneous groups we call "women" and "females." For those who menstruate, studies of the hormonal variation we experience throughout our menstrual cycles may lead to some changes in brain connectivity and ultimately behavior, but this may only be for *some women.* There are individual differences in behavioral hormone sensitivity; some women are supersensitive to hormonal changes while others breeze through their periods, pregnancy, and menopause without breaking a sweat. In the case of premenstrual syndrome (PMS), many studies have failed to prove that mood changes are driven by our menstrual cycle.[38] Some feminist writers go so far as to argue that PMS is a myth that reinforces the notion of the "hysterical female" with raging hormones.[39]

Other feminists challenge the way our medical system prioritizes mood-based PMS symptoms over physical symptoms, like pain and heavy bleeding. Period or pelvic pain is extremely common and known to have an effect on fatigue and other symptoms but is not included in PMS diagnostic criteria.[40] By pushing the "emotional female" agenda, the system has conveniently bypassed more rigorous research into what cyclical symptoms some women *do* experience and how they impact our mental health.

The problems may be in the science: studies measuring behavior and hormones are usually retrospective (asking participants to remember their symptoms), measured at a single time point, and self-reported, which could mean participants are telling researchers what they think they want to hear.[41] What the field really needs are studies that are longitudinal (gathering information over a long period, instead of at one time point), that are prospective (following participants over time instead of asking them to look backward), and that seek to determine within-person differences to help us discover whether some of us really are more sensitive to hormonal fluctuations than others. Anecdotally, I know a lot of my friends would strongly argue they are indeed sensitive to hormonal shifts in their bodies.

None of this research provides us with a clear answer to the question of whether women are more emotional, and if so, whether these emotions lead to more permanent states of moodiness. Of course, on any given day, a man might be more emotional or moodier than a woman. It depends largely on how the emotion is being measured and the situation in which it is being expressed.[42] What we can say is that there are likely some important gender differences in how emotions are learned, taught, and expressed. Even if science were able to prove that there are moderate sex or gender differences in our emotional lives, it wouldn't prove that this is how we've evolved as a species.[43]

Foundational studies in gender and emotion found that women have been socialized to express emotion differently from men. This research suggests that women feel and express more sadness, fear, and sympathy, whereas men feel and express more pride and anger.[44] However, these early studies used traditional methods in cognitive and emotion research, where photographs of adults' facial expressions were shown to participants (just like in picture books for toddlers with sad, happy, or scared faces), with the presumption that there are commonalities in emotional expression that all humans recognize. Anger is shown as a grimace, sadness as a frown, and happiness as a smile. But what if the idea of universal emotions doesn't hold true?

A MORE RECENT AND REVOLUTIONARY WAY to study and understand emotion stems from the idea that emotions are not triggered by a stimulus or limited to specific parts of the brain—emotions are *constructed* through our brain's complex network of neurons.[45] "In the case of Lisa Feldman Barrett, who was my graduate mentor... she was finding that people's experience of emotion was a mishmash," says Kristen Lindquist, professor of psychology and neuroscience at the University of North Carolina. "The brain evolved to make predictions about what the body needs in any given context. And so the brain is trying to keep the rest of the body alive... and making these predictions based on best guesses from prior experiences."

Lindquist says that at their core, emotions are biological and neurological states that help to keep our bodies in running order. It's our human language and culture that applies strict categories to emotion. "The basic notion of emotion in our particular culture comes with gendered baggage," says Lindquist. "You can see how the narrative of the emotional woman serves a purpose in certain societies to maintain power imbalances. And it becomes internalized by both men and women alike." When we grow up with the idea that women are emotional and men are not, our brain creates this gender bias in our everyday lived experience and in how we interact with each other.

I'm not suggesting here that the depression or anxiety you might be experiencing is made up. It is indeed very real! However, this area of research supports the idea that our culture has a strong influence on how our brain creates reality. If that's true, then Western culture's stereotype of the mentally ill woman could be part of what's driving up rates of depression and anxiety, almost like a self-fulfilling prophecy. Once we see that emotions are largely responses to our brain's need to keep us alive, we may be more successful in recognizing when our biased brains are setting us up to believe something that is not necessarily true. When doctors told me my broken brain was the cause of my mental illness, I believed them—at least until the treatments provided to me seemed to make matters worse. I then began to seek a different path to healing that considered the whole me (my biology and my gender) in relation to my social world.

GENDER BIAS IN THE DIAGNOSIS and treatment of women's mental illness medicalizes our bodies and pathologizes our emotions without providing appropriate support for the underlying issues at play. A lack of holistic care is never more apparent in a woman's life than during what I call the Big Three—adolescence, the perinatal period (pregnancy and postpartum), and menopause. We can experience mental health problems at other times in our lives, but these milestones come with significant hormonal changes and social stressors that, for some individuals, may trigger symptoms such as anxiety and depression. As this overview of gender bias shows us, multiple factors intermingle to create a sticky web that increases risk for mental health problems. When our bodies flip the switch during normal developmental periods of our lives, the results can be devastating.

3

BIOLOGY, HORMONES, AND MENTAL HEALTH

I do not think I ever opened a book in my life which had
not something to say upon woman's inconstancy. Songs
and proverbs, all talk of woman's fickleness. But perhaps
you will say, these were all written by men.

JANE AUSTEN'

FOR MANY YEARS, I understood my grandmother's mental
illness to be a genetic issue. A bad piece of DNA had infected
our family tree, and I was the next woman in line to feel its
effects. I found myself searching for evidence to prove that
narrative and trying to make sense of what it meant for my
grandmother, for me, and for my daughters.

It wasn't until I started mulling over the idea for this
book that I noticed an interesting pattern in our stories:
my grandmother was fifty when she started experiencing
the first signs of bipolar. I was sixteen when anxiety bull-
dozed my life. I was twenty-nine when I had my first child
and experienced postpartum mental illness. Each of those

occurrences coincides with a major reproductive transition in the life of a female.

A lightbulb went on. Could my grandmother's illness have been triggered by menopause? No doubt the gender-based stressors she experienced in her life—inequality, discrimination, abuse in the home, and trauma—had her balancing on a precipice. I wanted to know if it was hormonal changes that eventually pushed her over that ledge.

Before we dive in, I want to be clear: I don't think we need to reduce people to their reproductive or biological identities to study mental health. This is important to avoid, particularly for trans or nonbinary individuals, because biology is often used as means of discrimination. As I will repeat throughout this book, our mental health is determined by our biology, our lived experiences, and our environmental factors, all of which are influential in how we are supported and cared for in our communities. Women's overall well-being is much more than reproductive health, and evidence is scarce that genes *or* hormones play a starring role in anxiety and depression.[2] Not all women go through pregnancy and childbirth, so the hormone and brain changes that I cover in this chapter may not apply to you and your body. U.S. statistics show that in 2016, 14 percent of women between the ages of forty and forty-four didn't have children.[3]

All that said, sex hormones do influence female development, and it would be negligent of me to pass over this piece of the biopsychosocial trio. However, it's also important to acknowledge that not all women and girls find their mental health is affected by hormonal changes; as we saw in Chapter 2, certain individuals are more sensitive to developmental changes than others.[4]

When we analyze age and sex differences in rates of mental health disorders, Liisa Galea (whom you met in the last chapter) points to evidence that shows a higher prevalence during the female reproductive years.[5] "So that suggests to me some very strong biological components of that enhanced expression," she says.

When I tell her that I'm seeing a pattern in the stories women are sharing of their Big Three pivotal moments, she asks me what each of those life stages has in common. I stare at the screen, racking my brain for the right answer. Suddenly it feels like I'm back in a university lecture room, trying to answer a tough question from my professor.

"Um, they're all relevant to females?" I reply.

"Hormones!" she cries. "Puberty, pregnancy, postpartum, menopause—huge changes! That's why I'm studying hormones, because I think they're related."

Hormones regulate both our reproductive processes and our neural functioning, so they're pretty important for our bodies and brains.[6] Biologists have viewed these reproductive changes from an endocrine (hormonal) perspective, but neuroscience has revealed the complex interaction between the brain and our endocrine system.[7] Our bodies don't run the show—they're in an intricate dance with our brains, and the brain restructuring that occurs during significant shifts in our lives could hold clues as to why some of us are at a greater risk for mental health problems at these times. While puberty, pregnancy, and menopause are all reproductive transitions, they are also neurological processes.

To better understand how hormones affect our mental health, I needed a little primer on female hormones and what they do. Like many women, I was vaguely aware of this information, in a CliffsNotes kind of way. To learn more, I relied heavily on two books that are essential reading if you want to know more about reproductive transitions and mental health: Sarah McKay's *The Women's Brain Book: The Neuroscience of Health, Hormones, and Happiness*[8] and Jen Gunter's *The Menopause Manifesto: Own Your Health With Facts and Feminism.*[9]

Estrogen, progesterone, testosterone: you're probably familiar with the names of these hormones. When we discuss women's health, we often focus on estrogen. It was only when I delved into the research that I discovered that estrogen is not a single hormone: it's a grouping of three hormones called estradiol, estriol, and estrone. Estradiol and estrone are both primarily produced by the ovaries (estrone dominates after menopause), while estriol is made by the placenta during pregnancy. For the purposes of our discussion, the term "estrogen" will refer to the grouping of these three hormones.[10]

Estrogen is manufactured in the ovaries and brain, and it's vital to healthy brain function. For example, estrogen increases blood flow to the brain, enhances the brain's metabolism by increasing the efficiency of how it receives and uses chemicals, and helps to build strong communication in the neural pathways.[11] Estrogen also regulates the production of serotonin, an important neurotransmitter that is involved in mood regulation and memory (more on neurotransmitters in Chapter 9). When estrogen levels plummet after transitions like childbirth and menopause, the resulting drop in serotonin could be a factor in producing depressive or anxious symptoms.

But what I find even more interesting is that serotonin affects estrogen synthesis to bring us back to homeostasis.

This is a fancy word for how a system works to maintain stability even while experiencing changing conditions, and it's a necessary part of our survival.[12] It's like a sailor making continuous corrections so their ship does not get blown off course. Data shows that it may be a disruption of the relationship between estrogen and serotonin, and not a change in one or the other, that can elevate risk of mental health disorders.[13]

According to Galea, puberty, pregnancy, and menopause "are doing some structural changes to the brain... and so it's going to influence resiliency for sure." While these three transitions may put women more at risk of mental health problems, Galea isn't sure that the brain changes we see are necessarily risky. "They might even be better for you," she says.

For instance, research on brain changes that occur during adolescence shows that gray matter in the prefrontal cortex (the part of the brain that sits at the front of our skull) begins to thin. This is an important process of pruning unwanted neural connections in the brain, while the connections that remain are strengthened.[14] In pregnancy, brain volume changes may help us to feel more bonded to our babies.[15] And images of our brains during menopause have shown changes in brain structure, neural connectivity, and energy metabolism, which have the potential to make women more vulnerable to mental health issues *or* instead make us more resilient to change and better able to adapt.[16]

All these changes are likely serving a functional purpose, helping us transition into the next stage of life. Much more research is needed to determine what these brain changes mean and how social pressures related to gender at various stages in our lives interact with our biology and contribute to our overall risk of facing mental health challenges.

GIRLS AND YOUNG WOMEN

PERHAPS UNSURPRISINGLY, data from the Centers for Disease Control and Prevention shows that depression and anxiety are more common in teens than in young children. While we see more behavioral disorders and related diagnoses (attention-deficit/hyperactivity disorder, or ADHD, for example) for children aged six to eleven, diagnoses of anxiety and depression jump after the age of twelve.[17] What's more telling than prevalence are the patterns that have been observed over time: diagnoses of anxiety have increased over time, while diagnoses of depression have not changed. And once again, a gender gap appears, with higher rates of these mental health diagnoses in adolescent girls.

More recent global data suggests that the prevalence of anxiety and depression symptoms in teens during the COVID-19 pandemic *doubled* compared with life pre-pandemic, and these rates were higher in older adolescents and in girls.[18] Unfortunately, few studies in this analysis included youth from racialized communities or gender-diverse youth, who are at an increased risk of mental health issues. And as I reviewed in the last chapter, we also need to rely more on studies that track people over time, to see whether this high prevalence is sustained in the long term.

Even before the pandemic, researchers were sounding the alarm on the growing mental health crisis in adolescent girls. National Health Service (NHS) data from the U.K. in 2017 found that there were 17,500 instances of girls under seventeen admitted to the hospital for self-harm (for example, poisoning or cutting), a rise of 68 percent over the previous decade. So many girls were seeking help that there was concern the NHS child and adolescent mental health services would be overwhelmed.[19] Follow-up data from 2021 suggests that these numbers have worsened.[20]

It's important to note that this was self-reported data, which is not considered as reliable as more objective measures of mental distress (such as medical records). However, the outcomes the researchers reported are supported by many other studies performed worldwide, which reveal a pattern of increasing prevalence of mental health problems for adolescent girls.[21] A 2023 Canadian study shows a "marked and consistent" trend of rising suicide rates from 2000 to 2018 among adolescent females (ten to fourteen years) compared to stable rates in males.[22]

If we take a peek at brain and hormonal changes at this point in our lives, we can see the brain remodeling itself through the pruning of neural connections, the maturation of the stress-responsive regions in the brain, and drastic shifts in hormones.[23] Another big change is in how we learn to respond to stress. There are significant changes in the reactivity of our hypothalamic-pituitary-adrenal axis, which is a system that helps the body respond to stressors by regulating a number of our bodily functions (for example, our metabolism and immune response).[24] One way it does this is through the release of the primary stress hormone, cortisol.

In ancient times, our stressors were likely hungry predators and the threat of starvation, but in the modern world, a stressor could be a failing grade in school, a fight with our parents, or, more seriously, harassment or violence. Our brains respond in the same way they did all those moons ago when our greatest predators roamed the earth.

Stress is a part of life, and it's important to know that it's not bad for us to experience stress in general. However, adolescence is a time in life when we are experiencing many different types of stressors, and simultaneously our bodies are changing how we respond to that stress. When hormones shift, the body's stress response can be either over-activated or underactivated, and it appears that girls' (and women's) cortisol responses are *lower* than boys' and men's during times of stress.[25] Since cortisol's job is to help our bodies deal with stressful situations, an underactive cortisol response may lead to a higher risk of depression following a stressful experience.[26] This is likely because parts of the female brain remain on high alert following stress rather than heading back to a calmer state.

Beyond biology, what else has been going on for teen girls that could exacerbate mental health issues? Think "social." Facebook launched in 2004 as an online social network where students could judge the attractiveness of their peers. The people responsible for engineering social media (and essentially our social lives as we now know them) promoted a design with the ability to rank people and the data they were sharing by popularity.[27] Instagram was launched a few years later, in 2010, followed by an avalanche of other social apps, all designed to suck us into a system that relies on algorithmic ranking of the latest shiny thing. If you're interested in reading further on this, Johann Hari's analysis of the history and design of social media in his book *Stolen Focus: Why You Can't Pay Attention—and How to Think Deeply Again* is excellent.[28]

The online world was in its infancy when I first experienced mental health problems as a teen, so it had no impact on my own journey. But I have two young girls approaching their teen years and know firsthand some of the problems they face. Heavy social media use is associated with depressive symptoms in adolescent girls more than it is in adolescent boys. If we go back to the causes of the gender gap in mental health disorders that I outlined from *The Lancet*, you might remember that women's lower self-esteem and higher risk for body-related shame may be implicated in the higher rates of mental illness in women. It appears that social media, which research has linked to body image dissatisfaction and lower self-esteem, compounds these risks.[29]

Body image and self-esteem problems are associated with internalizing symptoms—meaning individuals are more likely to turn their distress inward—such as excessive worry, headaches or digestive issues, anxiety, and depression. Research on sex differences linked to these symptoms shows that internalizing is more prevalent in females compared with males.[30] The theory is that when the female threat-stress response is activated, it's sometimes not able to turn off again to help the body recover. As we've seen, females tend to have an underactivated response in the *moment* of stress and struggle to shut off the response well after the threat has departed. This may be why females fall more into rumination, because we have longer periods of time between facing a threat and reaching an eventual recovery stage.[31]

Essentially, social media may be fuel for the fire—if girls and women were *already* more likely to struggle with body shame and low self-esteem prior to Instagram and Snapchat, the fuel of the feed has turned our small fire into an inferno.

Social challenges in the adolescent years can occur beyond the bright glow of our smartphone screens, but it could be that the way we interact online complicates this normal process of development. Teenage girls often seek out a new tribe as they grow from children into adults, moving toward more independence and control over their own lives.[32] This is an essential step in a teen's brain growth and development, but since much of our social world now takes place through online interactions, it is more difficult for parents to monitor issues of cyberbullying, which appear to disproportionately affect teen girls.[33]

The answer to these problems may not be banning social media for teen girls but rather targeting specific factors that increase the risk of developing anxiety and depression. This includes measures to prevent and target cyberbullying; to help teen girls achieve better-quality sleep (maybe by turning off Wi-Fi at night or using monitoring systems to shut down apps); and to improve well-being through more physical activity.[34] Later in the book, I'll review strategies that may help girls to manage their stress responses through the process of embodiment. By turning our attention away from screens for periods of time and learning how to tap into the body, we can recognize and better manage stress.

THE FINAL PIECE of the adolescent mental health puzzle, which is, in my opinion, the most crucial, is the way in which our culture exerts its influence over the female body. This influence is twofold and contradictory: on one hand, girls are taught that menstruating bodies are dirty and shameful and that we should keep a tight lid on the emotional whirlwind of puberty. A great illustration is in the 2022 Disney and Pixar film *Turning Red*, in which a young teen girl named Mei Lee turns into a giant red panda whenever her emotions get the better of her—an entertaining metaphor for puberty and menstruation. Mei navigates her family's expectation that she will give up her red panda identity, just as other women in the family have done. The reaction to the film provided a second lesson: it received countless online reviews warning parents that the themes were too mature and overly sexualized, and that the movie's Chinese-Canadian character was unrelatable.[35] The story happily flouts societal expectations of what girls are supposed to think and feel and how they are supposed to act, which clearly touched a nerve.

While girls are internalizing this discourse on modesty and control, they're also hearing conflicting cultural messages that their bodies are the object of sexual desire and attention. In 2019, the research organization NORC at the University of Chicago conducted a two-thousand-person survey in the U.S., which found that 81 percent of women and 43 percent of men reported experiencing some form of sexual harassment or sexual assault in their lifetime.[36] This included verbal harassment, unwanted touching, cyber harassment, being followed, genital flashing, and sexual assault. Many of us have likely found the courage to share our #MeToo stories thanks to founder Tarana Burke's indefatigable work. What's illuminating about the mounting evidence of widespread sexual harassment and abuse of women is that we know that repeated stressors in childhood and adolescence can affect brain development and stress response. Sexual harassment and abuse in adolescence directly contribute to women's mental and physical health challenges, making us vulnerable to ongoing psychiatric problems.[37] We will do a deep dive into this topic in Chapter 6.

Given the high rates of mental health problems in adolescence and the difficulties girls encounter when seeking treatment, it's possible that these mental health issues spill over into young adulthood. Even if women are finally able to get a handle on things, they may soon be entering a different transition altogether: one of rapid physical and hormonal shifts, sleep troubles, and hundreds of diaper changes. And one that society tells us is the most important job we'll ever do (no pressure, though).

PREGNANCY AND POSTPARTUM

PATRICIA TOMASI IS COFOUNDER of the Canadian Perinatal Mental Health Collaborative, the first and only advocacy organization calling on the federal government to enact a national perinatal mental health strategy.

As with many women, Patricia's story began in adolescence when she experienced panic attacks, anxiety, and depression. Emergency department doctors and her family doctor identified her symptoms as anxiety or panic, but no proper support or treatment was ever provided. "No one ever told me that I would be at a higher risk of developing prenatal or postpartum mental health issues because of my history of mental health," she says.

After she became pregnant with her first child, her symptoms escalated throughout the pregnancy and worsened after the birth. "I didn't want to see the baby—I just wanted to be left alone," she recalls. "I couldn't sleep, had extreme anxiety, palpitations, muscle tightness, panic." No one screened her for mental health issues at postpartum checkups, and the advice she received was to eat well and sleep. "If I had really mild prenatal and postpartum anxiety and depression, maybe eating well and trying to sleep might have helped a little bit. But I was on the moderate to severe end. I needed to be hospitalized," she says.

Patricia's illness worsened over time, and she had her first manic episode six months after the birth. "I started to get into spirituality, and I thought angels were talking to me," she says. "We lost our house because I thought angels were telling me to quit my job and become a hands-on energy healer." And still, because she was in no danger of harming herself or her baby, she didn't receive any help from medical professionals.

Then came a second pregnancy, and Patricia suspects that something in her shifting hormones helped her mood to stabilize. She gained a sense of perspective on her experiences from her previous pregnancy and postpartum and was incredulous that the situation had spiraled so far out of control. Yet Patricia says, "I still thought it was something that I could control, that I had brought it on myself."

She focused on taking care of herself throughout her second pregnancy: eating well, doing yoga, and taking hypnobirthing classes. She received midwifery care, after having had obstetrical care for her first pregnancy, so she had access to more one-on-one attention. Her marriage was strong, and she didn't have outside stress. "Everything was 'perfect,'" she says, lifting her hands to make air quotes.

But after she gave birth, the symptoms returned—only ten times worse. "Then a lightbulb went off and I went, 'How could this be happening? If everything's okay on the outside?'" she says. The realization hit that what she was experiencing was a biologically based illness and something that she couldn't control on her own.

Even then, Patricia had to take charge and request treatment. "I only got medication because I went in ... and demanded that my family doctor run the Edinburgh Postnatal Depression Scale," she says. "And my score wasn't that high, because my symptoms were more anxiety, and that scale tends to lean more toward depression." Still, she persevered, watching her doctor look up the evidence on which mental health medications would be safe to take while breastfeeding. There were no follow-up appointments booked to discuss the medication's efficacy or side effects. "I had to direct my own medical care," she says.

"Pregnancy and postpartum," says Galea, "do create a perfect storm for mental health disorders, because we see the same kind of biomarkers occurring during those stages that we see in mental health problems." In depression, there is a reduction in volume of the hippocampus, a part of the brain that's involved in memory and the weaving together of separate events into a single narrative.[38] As Galea points out, the *same reduction* occurs in pregnancy and postpartum. Other major changes in the perinatal period affect our immune system, stress hormones, and metabolism—all in ways similar to what we see during an episode of major depression. "So maybe it's not that surprising that there's an increased risk, right?" says Galea. "The issue is how do you mitigate against that increased risk?"

The antidepressant medication Patricia started worked wonders, and after five to six weeks, her symptoms started to resolve. After three months, she felt like herself again. "I felt normal—no anxiety, no depression, no panic, no constant worrying, no racing thoughts, no intrusive thoughts. I just felt so good." She was asked to blog about her postpartum anxiety journey for *HuffPost Canada*, and with her background in journalism, she also wrote about the state of maternal mental health in Canada. She interviewed top experts from across the country and around the world and quickly noticed a significant gap in the system. "I was like, 'Where are the advocates? Who's changing this?'" she says.

"It's impossible to get funding," says Galea, when we talk about the research field of perinatal mood disorders. "It's a very heterogeneous disorder, because not everyone that gets perinatal depression has the same kind of symptoms and some women are more susceptible to hormonal changes than others." This is why female-only studies are essential to building our knowledge around reproductive transitional phases and women's mental health: they give us a sense of disease progress and outcomes *as they relate to females.* "I want to know, in females, how does this work differently... depending on my age, my experience, or how many children I've had," says Galea.

To her point, mental illness in the perinatal period is influenced by more than just biology, and there are multiple social factors that pressure mothers in Western society to perform to certain standards (which we'll cover more in Chapter 7).

But what is likely an even bigger issue in North America is the lack of a social safety net. Though Canada offers twelve to eighteen months of paid parental leave, American mothers have no national paid parental leave program, and only 21 percent of U.S. workers have access to paid family leave through their employers.[39] In Canada, there are disparities between "parental leave rich" and "parental leave poor" families, with some parents who don't qualify for benefits or don't receive top-ups from employers.[40] The research is mounting that shows countries that invest heavily in paid family leave have happier and healthier parents (and, by extension, happier children).[41]

TO EXPLORE THE IMPORTANCE of this social safety net, I sat down with Lola, a friend who kindly offered to share her story with me. She doesn't remember any significant mental health concerns in her teen years but says that things got bad when she became pregnant shortly after the death of her mother. "I had massive anxiety during my pregnancy," she says, "and I was sleeping only two to three hours a night, maximum."

After her baby was born, she remembers that much of her anxiety was funneled into worries about the health of the baby and the risk of sudden infant death syndrome (SIDS). To make matters worse, her newborn cried most of the day and didn't sleep at night, adding to Lola's sleep deprivation.

"We have nobody, which is just so difficult," she says, when I ask her what she thinks was the main cause of her postpartum anxiety. "When you're going to have a baby and you have no family to help, it's really, really hard." But she adds that the lack of sleep was likely the biggest culprit. Research on the relationship between sleep and postpartum mental disorders backs this up (although findings are mixed due to some poor-quality studies).[42] However, culture has a lot to do with sleep quality. In a review of traditional postpartum practices and rituals, the authors found that some cultures provide organized support to new mothers, including prescribed periods of rest, and these practices are thought to protect and restore women's health, often through nourishing food and proper sleep.[43]

"Fixing" infants' and mothers' sleep is a huge obsession in North America, and you can't have a baby these days without being given one of the hundreds of books on infant sleep training—whether it prescribes a "gentle" method or a "cry it out" technique. There are also sleep trainers galore, and many high-income families fork out hundreds of dollars to get support for their baby's sleep. However, this hyperfocus on sleep is likely not getting to the heart of the problem, which is that many families (like Lola's) are parenting without a solid social safety net. Though Lola's partner shouldered the burden of cooking, cleaning, and taking care of Lola, they were both lacking support from extended family and other community members.

In Lola's case, the sleep issue fixed itself, until baby number two came along and the whole process started again. Following the birth of her second child, Lola lost her full-time job and went back to school to upgrade her qualifications. During this job upheaval and the pressures of raising a young family, Lola entered menopause at the age of forty-seven. Her story is an interesting case of two transitional periods colliding.

MENOPAUSE

MEDICAL LITERATURE CALLS menopause the "menopausal transition," which is said to begin when our menstrual periods become irregular and end with our last period. There are hormonal, biological, and clinical features that indicate menopause has started, but most women notice irregular cycles, heavier periods, and other physiological symptoms, like hot flashes. Perimenopause, another term used in the literature, marks the transitional time between cycle irregularity and up to one year after a woman's final period. It's a broader term that encompasses the sometimes lengthy process of change we go through in midlife, from pre- to postmenopause.[44] Hormonally, perimenopause is characterized by a big drop in estrogen, which is why it's sometimes called our "second puberty" or "reverse puberty."

In *The Menopause Manifesto*, author and gynecologist Jen Gunter writes that menopause is often conceived of as a process of ovarian failure, a disease that affects women because our ovaries are weak. (Sound familiar?) The basis for this argument is that men don't experience menopause. "Comparing women and men in this way is the same as comparing the liver with the heart. The liver isn't weak or diseased because it doesn't beat like the heart," she writes.[45]

Longitudinal studies have shown that women are at a significantly increased risk of developing depression in perimenopause and postmenopause, measured either through a symptom inventory—a scale or checklist—or in structured clinical interviews.[46] Depending on the study, women's risk for depression around menopause is reported as anywhere from 19 percent to 36 percent.[47] These results are based on just a few studies, and you won't be surprised to learn that research on the link between menopause and mood is lacking. There are very few studies that compare women in different menopausal stages, so we have little understanding of how mood disorders may be different in each stage and how they change over time. In addition, while cross-sectional studies in different parts of the world show an increased risk for

depression in menopause, more studies are needed to clarify this risk for different ethnic, racial, and cultural groups.

"I was raging," says Lola. "My partner had never seen me
like that—I was so angry." Lola feels that hormones were
likely part of the problem, but she thought that the rage was
more a symptom of her anxiety. "And maybe a lack of feeling
supported," she says. "Being bitter that we can't just leave
the kids with Grandma and Grandpa and go do something."

It's difficult to tease apart what happens to our mental
health in menopause. As always, it appears to be a combination of physiological, medical, social, and psychological
factors that create the perfect storm for mental problems. Science tells us that changes in our body's estrogen levels affect
how other neural pathways function, including our body
temperature, libido, sleep, emotions, attention, and memory.[48]
And most of us would recognize that lack of sleep, difficulty
concentrating, and loss of sex drive can trigger low mood.

Further to this, estrogen is thought to moderate serotonin
and dopamine levels, which affect mood, memory, and the
experience of pleasure.[49] However, the exact mechanisms
by which menopause alters brain physiology to generate
these symptoms is unclear. What we do know is that menopause is not a *cause* of depression, but hormonal shifts trigger
symptoms and some women are more sensitive to the drop
in estrogen than others.[50]

After she started taking an antidepressant, Lola remembers her symptoms of anxiety and rage abating, but she still
wasn't feeling like herself. "I went to my doctor, and I'm
like, 'I want a referral to a psychiatrist.' And my doctor said,
'Listen, Lola, everybody and their brother are depressed and
have anxiety right now... It's going to take a really, really

long time to get in.'" He asked Lola how long it had been since she was in menopause and whether she'd ever tried hormone replacement therapy, or HRT.

"I was always under the impression that it wasn't good for you, and that it was better to be natural," she says. This misconception, still widely held, stems from results of the Women's Health Initiative (WHI) study in 2002, which showed that HRT could increase the risk of heart disease and breast cancer. The results were splashed across popular media, women and doctors panicked, and most people stopped prescribing and taking hormones.

The results of the WHI, though, were controversial. Most participants in the trial were more than ten years past their final menstrual period, which meant the results couldn't be applied to younger women. A reanalysis of the trial a decade later showed that the use of HRT in younger women and those within ten years of the start of menopause had *better* cardiovascular outcomes.[51] The risk of breast cancer was found to be very small overall, and for some women, the benefits of HRT for treating symptoms of menopause may outweigh the slightly increased breast cancer risk.

Lola was thrilled to find that HRT worked well for treating her psychological symptoms. She felt better able to focus on herself and was soon set to start therapy for the first time.

MENOPAUSE IS AS MUCH a social and psychological transition as it is a hormonal one, and there are other important psychosocial risk factors. Trauma and violence against women can lead to long-term stress because of chronically elevated levels of the hormone cortisol.[52] Over time, high cortisol levels can have a significant negative impact on our brain function. One study that followed 682 women for almost two decades found that a history of sexual abuse was associated with worse menopausal symptoms and worse general health.[53] As I read this paper, I reflected on the years of emotional abuse my grandmother experienced, the financial insecurity she faced with a husband who drank all their money, and the trauma of losing her firstborn child to scarlet fever when he was only two years old. Popular culture is now well versed in the language of trauma, and many of us better understand its influence on our mental health, but I feel a deep sadness that my grandmother was never held and supported in the ways she needed to be.

Decreased social support and negative attitudes toward aging and femininity in Western culture have also been shown to play a role in mood disorders during the menopausal transition. (In many other cultures, people respect and celebrate their elders, across genders.) It's been found that women with more negative attitudes to menopause report more physical and emotional symptoms.[54] And these negative attitudes stem from cultural messaging that tells us that everything about aging as a woman is wrong. In her book *Navigating the Messy Middle*, author Ann Douglas shares stories from more than one hundred women in midlife, stories that underscore two competing narratives about menopause. One is the narrative of decline—that women have reached their peak and it's all downhill from here. This story is part of the negative attitude toward aging that could affect our well-being; we're told that we're "old news" and no longer worthy of attention. Celebrity culture is rife with women who feel they've been passed over once they reach a certain age.

The flip side is the successful aging story, where women are told that midlife will be the time of their lives, full of positive transformation and freedom. But for women who reach menopause and face financial challenges, disability, or loss, the reality is—as Douglas says—messy.[55] However, she argues that there is much meaning to be found in the diversity of women's individual experiences. "When our midlife narratives are too limited and too limiting, we end up feeling like we're invisible or that we've failed," she writes.[56] I feel cautiously optimistic in seeing menopause being talked about more openly among my peers (although, yes, we still have a trail to blaze), and sharing the diversity of our experiences can set us up for more realistic expectations and a healthier transition.

WHAT'S THE GOOD NEWS?

I KNOW I'VE PAINTED a bleak picture of women's mental health over our life span. But fear not, there is good news *and* there are also promising treatments and social supports that can make a real difference in our lives. I did find this tidbit encouraging: most women undergoing menopause do not experience long-term adverse effects, and I would suspect that the same could be said for other transitional times in our lives.[57] Although some of us may be vulnerable to the hormonal and neurological shifts during the Big Three, a culture of strong support alongside effective treatment can interrupt the repetitive cycle of mental problems.

And here's another piece of good news: preclinical studies have shown that our brain can compensate for the drop in estrogen we experience during menopause.[58] In fact, we develop this ability to compensate over our whole lives, as we experience changes in gray and white matter, in neural connectivity, and in brain energy consumption (how much glucose the brain uses). "Women's brains also have a unique plasticity," writes Jen Gunter, "the ability to change or rewire in response to hormonal cues," which is a logical and necessary neurological mechanism that helps us to prepare for major life transitions.[59] In adolescence, one of our tasks is to pull away from family and form our own social tribe. In pregnancy, our brain shifts its precious resources to the vital task of keeping our fetus growing. In menopause, the brain goes through significant remodeling as our reproductive time comes to an end; it learns to compensate and adapt to a new normal. The brain knows how to recover.

Could it be possible that women's brains are functioning just as they should throughout all development stages of our lives? I'm not suggesting that mental illness during these time points is normal, or that we should just embrace that it's happening. I'm arguing that a healthier environment— one that fosters girls' and women's well-being—could better support our transitioning brains. More robust data, better-quality treatments, and community-based resources could be the ticket to assist women throughout these transitions, reducing the risk that mental health problems become serious, chronic illnesses.

Donna Jackson Nakazawa, author of *Girls on the Brink: Helping Our Daughters Thrive in an Era of Increased Anxiety, Depression, and Social Media*, writes: "A neuroprotective environment is one in which the conditions that foster a sense of being safely seen, deeply connected, and valued have been set in place by parents and other family members, mentors, and community. Each of these neuroprotective spheres of influence lies nestled inside the next, larger sphere, as with a series of Matryoshka dolls, each painted wooden doll held inside the next. If we are to grow strong girls, each neuro-protective sphere must pass the litmus test of whether girls feel secure and connected within it."[60]

Let's not stop at adolescence, though. As a society, we have a communal responsibility to foster safety and con-nection for women at all stages of their life. To accomplish this, we have a lot of work to do to change the systems we so urgently depend on.

4

WHAT'S TRULY BROKEN?
HOW MENTAL HEALTH
CARE HAS FAILED
WOMEN

Ideal mental health, like freedom, exists for
one person only if it exists for all people.
PHYLLIS CHESLER[1]

MY YOUNG ADULT LIFE was a master class in faking it. From
the outside, things looked good. Early intervention and therapy (which I'll get into in more detail in Chapter 8) made a
big difference in my life, and I started university without any
major hiccups. But mental illness was a burdensome secret,
and it felt that at any moment the ground would give way
under my feet.

And, sure enough, it did. I relapsed in my second year
of university and missed my final exams; I went through
a humiliating process of getting a doctor's note to explain

why I needed to defer my finals. I was relieved to see the note was vague, and I lied to my classmates and professors that what I had was a physical illness. When pressed for details, I would say "stomach problems" and scrunch up my nose to ward off any follow-up questions. No one wants to hear about digestive issues.

After finishing my exams over the summer, I did what many young people do in a crisis: I fled. I transferred all my credits to a different university, packed up, and moved several hours away. If I'd been in therapy at the time, I suspect my therapist would have reminded me that running away is not usually the best solution to our problems. But I'd aged out of child mental health services and struggled to find someone I could work with over the long term. Despite having significant advantages (supportive parents and financial stability being two biggies), I still felt lost navigating a system that seemed as broken as I imagined myself to be.

LONG WAIT TIMES for services, lack of access to effective treatments, and enduring stigma about mental illness are global problems. The solutions need to be grounded in the knowledge that mental illness affects twice as many women as men, and that bias exists in every facet of the medical system. More importantly, though, women are not all the same—we come from different cultures and socioeconomic backgrounds, and we have different lived experiences, such as those related to sexual and physical violence, caregiving roles, and barriers to equality.

Even when women have the financial means and motivation to seek help, they are often shunted around to different medical specialists, dismissed as being simply "stressed out," or handed a prescription and sent on their way. For other women, the system in which they could seek care is inadequate, due to lack of insurance, lack of culturally competent health care providers, and/or mental illness stigma, which is often greater among marginalized populations.[2] It's clearly time for a new strategy—one that tackles system-level disparities, while offering individualized approaches to care.

ACCESS DENIED: BARRIERS
TO MENTAL HEALTH CARE

IF WE THINK about mental health care in basic economic terms, there are supply and demand sides of the system. (Later, I'll discuss a different and better way to approach the system.) Demand for mental health services has increased around the world, but supply has largely remained the same or has even decreased in some areas.

High demand in Western countries has far outpaced supply, leading to serious waitlist problems. The challenge in finding accurate data on this is that many countries don't track national wait times, leaving researchers to try to fill in the gap:

- In Canada in 2021, individuals waited up to one month for counseling services, with one in ten people waiting more than four months.[3] In my home province of Ontario, a 2020 report found that children and youth under eighteen were waiting as long as two and a half *years* to receive mental health treatment, with waitlists doubling in the previous two years.[4]

- In the United States, anecdotal evidence suggests that some patients are waiting an average of five to six weeks for both private and community-based services,[5] and many are unable to find a private therapist with space available.[6]

- In a poll conducted by the Royal College of Psychiatrists in the U.K. (where wait times can be long), it was found that a "hidden waitlist" kept 65 percent of patients waiting more than four weeks between their initial intake appointment and follow-up appointment; 23 percent of people were waiting for more than three months.[7]

I did find some bright spots. Many countries within the European Union have targets for wait times and aim to provide treatment or first point of contact within one to three months. Some Nordic countries (Denmark, Finland, Norway, and Estonia) have increased the percentage of people being seen within nationally set wait times, or by a deadline based on the individual's clinical assessment (Norway).[8] In these countries, wait times have improved mainly thanks to "supply-side policies"—increasing the number of care providers or expanding the scope of care—rather than taming the increased demand.

In my own country, the supply of mental health services continues to fall short of demand. In 2018, around 5.3 million Canadians had expressed a need for help for their mental health issues in the past year.[9] Of these, 1.2 million (22 percent) said that their needs were only partially met and 1.1 million (21 percent) said that their needs were fully unmet. The most frequently reported reasons for having partially or fully unmet needs were: lack of knowledge about where to find services, being too busy, or not being able to afford to pay out of pocket. Very similar data exists for the U.S., where in 2018, 39 percent of people cited cost as the top reason for unmet treatment needs, although that number had declined from 45 percent in 2008.[10] Of note, three other reasons patients gave for unmet needs in this survey—"thinking they could handle the problem without treatment," "didn't know where to go for treatment," and "did not have time"—all showed an increased number of responses since 2008. Notably, over 22 percent of people from the Canadian "unmet needs" groups reported that they preferred to manage their mental health on their own. The need that was most likely to be met was for medication (85 percent), while the need for therapy was most likely to be unmet (34 percent).[11]

As we improve awareness of mental health and reduce stigma, more people are recognizing when they're struggling, but that doesn't mean they always have the knowledge, motivation, resources, or time to seek help. This flags another problem with access: we place responsibility on the individual to research their own treatment options and navigate the system with little decision-making support. In my own country, a diagnosis of physical illness results in a swift and efficient entry into a system that coordinates your care; it may still be confusing and difficult at times, but the infrastructure is there to ensure you get timely and focused access to treatment. Mental health care really has no "system"; there is a complete lack of coordinated care.[12]

It's common knowledge among researchers and clinicians that the earlier an individual receives an intervention, the more likely their mental health crisis will be resolved through a brief stint of talk therapy. This makes it less likely that someone will depend on medication over the long term or resort to visits to the emergency room to access care.[13] As we'll cover in Chapter 9, medication can be a positive and welcome part of a mental health treatment plan; however, many people prefer not to be on medication, and face difficult side effects and trouble coming off the drugs when the crisis is over. When medications are used in place of talk therapy due to long wait times or financial barriers, individuals are not provided the opportunity to tackle the underlying problem or develop the necessary skills to promote healing and resiliency.[14]

Who can afford it?

IN THE CONTEXT OF WESTERN COUNTRIES, mental health services are not available to all, in terms of both accessibility and affordability. In the U.S. medical system, policy disparities exist between mental and general health care. Medicaid, the health coverage provided to millions of low-income Americans, excludes reimbursement for many inpatient psychiatric care facilities.[15] Payments for outpatient care also trail behind other medical specialties, and there are fewer psychiatrists who take insurance compared to physicians in other specialties.[16] Psychiatrists receive lower insurance rates for their services compared to other medical or surgical physicians.[17] This is a disappointing outcome given a federal law passed in 2008 that required most insurance companies to cover mental health services comparably to physical health services.[18]

While there are some government-funded services (free for the user) for mental health, including a new three-digit dialing code for suicide prevention and services at community mental health centers, more than one-third of Americans live in "health workforce shortage areas," where there are not enough mental health providers to cover population needs.[19] In 2022, the Biden administration announced millions of dollars in grants to expand all-hours mental health and substance use care through community clinics, a welcome injection of funds to programs that had historically received spotty financial support.[20] Community clinic programs are unique in that they care for those with mental illness close to home, which helps patients avoid traveling long distances to larger centers or inpatient units.[21]

My own country's health care system operates similarly to those in Australia and the U.K. Though Canadians like to pat ourselves on the back for addressing some of the financial barriers to physical health care, when it comes to mental health, there are still striking gaps. One article states that in 2013, 30 percent of Canadians who see private-practice psychotherapists pay out of pocket, a collective total of $950 million annually.[22] In the U.K., *The Guardian* reports that in 2022 the NHS was paying two billion pounds per year to private hospitals to care for mental health patients due to a shortage of beds in public hospitals. The same research found that independent mental health care providers had 91 percent of their income paid by the NHS.[23]

I've been paying out of pocket for private therapy for over three years, and other than the provincially funded care I received as a child, most of my adult therapists have been minimally covered by workplace benefits and wellness programs. The quality of these services has varied greatly, and it's only in the past decade that I've had the financial means to access a therapist I feel connected to and who offers a therapeutic approach that is highly effective for me (but I'm still paying out of pocket).

My financial position has dictated where (and when) I can access therapy. In the past, I've also faced barriers related to transportation options and costs, economic costs from missed work, and often a lack of choice—both of provider and of the frequency of contact with my therapist. As research shows, all of the barriers that exist when it comes to mental health services are compounded by gender disparities.

Gender-specific barriers to care

WOMEN OF REPRODUCTIVE AGE (generally defined as those aged fifteen to forty-nine, with or without children) have high rates of contact with the health care system yet continue to experience unmet needs for mental health care. One survey found that thirteen million reproductive-aged women in the U.S. had severe or moderate psychological distress. Compared with women who reported no psychological distress, they were more likely to experience delayed health care or no care, with cost identified as the greatest barrier. Other reasons for delayed care included: "couldn't get through on phone," "couldn't get appointment soon enough," and "wait too long in doctor's office."[24] Women with children need to juggle childcare and household management, of which they are responsible for a greater proportion even when they have partners.

For older women, there is a lack of research on access to mental health services and mental health outcomes, because data often lumps all older women into the sixty-five-plus category. The health concerns of a woman at sixty-five might be very different from her needs at ninety. Without disaggregating data by sex *and* age, the needs of older women remain invisible.[25]

This is concerning, given that women generally live longer than men, suffer more from chronic or complex health issues, and are more likely to be caregivers for children or elderly parents.[26] Some data suggests that the gender disadvantage women face when it comes to their mental health continues into old age, despite earlier research that showed that women are less affected by mental health issues after the menopausal transition.[27] Other challenges that may impact access to care and that disproportionately affect older women include financial strain, limited mobility, transportation, and street safety.[28] (Young women are also more greatly affected by these issues compared to men of the same age.) For women of all ages who live in rural areas, transportation is vital to access health care, as distances to care providers are usually greater and there are fewer modes of transportation.

Women with disabilities face unique hurdles in accessing mental health care. As with other underrepresented groups, there is a general lack of existing data and knowledge on the needs of women with disabilities, but studies show that they face a greater risk of interpersonal violence, discrimination, and barriers in making informed health decisions (because they may not receive accessible information), along with higher rates of poverty. In addition, their transportation costs can be much higher than for women without disabilities, and there are additional structural barriers, such as lack of accessible clinic entrances, elevators, or other supportive equipment, as well as communication barriers with health care providers.[29]

Not all of these challenges can be addressed by throwing more money or mental health providers at the problem. Solutions need to account for the fact that many women with mental health problems may be least able to navigate the system because of gender-specific disadvantages and discrimination. Women need supportive workplace policies, easier access to childcare options, financial support, and other social safety nets—all designed to make it easier for us to get the care we desire, when we want and need it.

KATHERINE'S SEVERE DEPRESSION and suicidal ideation began at the age of twelve and culminated in a suicide attempt. "It was a cry for help," as one doctor described it to her, and Katherine now agrees. "It definitely was," she says.

Thanks to her mother's connections at a local hospital, Katherine was referred to a child psychologist. She remembers a single intake session with no follow-up, but she did start seeing a social worker at school. Her mental health improved until she reached early adulthood, when the depression returned. Finding the treatment she needed to get better was a challenge, as was accessing a long enough stint of therapy. "A lot of times, you can get like six sessions for free and then you're cut off," she says. "My problems cannot be solved in six sessions."

She remembers one time in particular: "I had an intake with a psychologist ... and it was like, 'Finally, I've spoken to someone.' But then I'm waiting and waiting and waiting." There was no follow-up after her initial intake appointment; after one month, she called the center back and was informed that they had a long waitlist of patients. "And basically it felt like because I wasn't actively suicidal, I could wait." Katherine was finally offered a handful of sessions from a social worker, whose approach to treatment veered into toxic positivity—a belief that no matter how difficult a situation is, optimism and positivity are all you need to get through it. "Her attitude basically seemed to be 'Don't worry, be happy,' and I was like, 'Lady, if I could do that, I wouldn't be here,'" Katherine says. Her mom eventually chose to pay out of pocket for Katherine to see a private psychologist, an option that's not available to many women.

Katherine wishes that people didn't have to show up at the emergency room having attempted suicide in order to access proper help. "I feel like it shouldn't have to get to that point," she says. "What would our society look like if we could get to people before they reach that point?" Six sessions might help some people, and it's better than nothing, but Katherine asks, "Is that where the bar is—'It's better than nothing'?"

Katherine feels that for her, the issue with access to services has been less about her identity as a woman and more about Canada's lack of resources and the need to pay out of pocket for therapy. "If you have money, you can see someone tomorrow; if you don't have money, good luck," she says. "I'm [currently] seeing a psychotherapist and not a psychologist partly because she's cheaper. She does a great job, but also I cannot afford to see a psychologist."

With cost and access as significant barriers, it's important to remember that research shows that gender influences socioeconomic status. Women have higher rates of poverty compared to men and are disproportionately represented in jobs that are low paying and more precarious.[30] In the U.S., these issues are experienced to a greater degree by American

Indian or Alaska Native women, Black women, and Latinas. In Canada in 2021, 11.4 percent of women were living in low-income households compared to 9.7 percent of men.[31] Gender is indeed the common denominator here, and tackling issues of poverty and financial strain requires targeted approaches for different groups of women.

"Women tend to [be] the center of the family," says psychiatrist Cornelia Wieman, acting chief medical officer at the First Nations Health Authority in British Columbia and past president of the Indigenous Physicians Association of Canada. In her work with Indigenous women, Wieman observes that many don't have partners or are co-parenting but not living with partners. "That prevents women, in some cases, from seeking services in the first place; there's no childcare options," she says.

Wieman can recall times she's tried to do a psychiatric assessment for a woman whose three children are running around the exam room, knocking everything over. "It's not really amenable to an actual assessment," she says. For a woman with substance use problems, a residential program may be the best option for care, but Wieman knows that her patient doesn't have reliable childcare options. "They're kind of stuck between a rock and a hard place of trying to look after their health but not being able to access certain services."

As a biracial woman, Katherine is also facing stigma from within her own family and culture. Her dad is Indian, from Punjab, where there is significant shame tied to mental illness and therapy. "When it comes to therapy, that means you're crazy; it means you're an embarrassment," she says. "[Our culture doesn't] do therapy." Katherine's situation is not unique, and many women find that when they try to access mental health services, the people providing care sometimes don't understand their cultural or ethnic identities.

MIND THE GAP: RACISM AND DIVERSITY IN MENTAL HEALTH CARE

NORTH AMERICA IS HOME to an increasingly diverse population. The American Psychiatric Association estimates that by 2044, more than half of all Americans will belong to a group other than non-Hispanic white. Around nine million adults in the United States identify as lesbian or gay, bisexual, or transgender (though survey numbers vary widely).[32] We also know that socioeconomic status, race, and ethnicity are intimately intertwined, in that race and ethnicity often influence someone's income, educational attainment, and financial security.[33]

The lack of racial and ethnic diversity in the U.S. psychiatric workforce contrasts starkly with America's growing diversity. A recent study on psychiatric physicians did a comparison: 10.4 percent of practicing psychiatrists are underrepresented minorities in medicine compared with 32.6 percent in the entire U.S. population; 38.5 percent of psychiatrists are women compared with 50.8 percent of the U.S. population. It's clear that there's a bit of a mismatch between those providing care and those needing care.[34]

Survey rates of depression among racial and ethnic groups in the U.S. have mixed findings, and some data shows lower depression rates in Asian and Afro-Caribbean immigrants compared to American-born whites.[35] Another survey published in 2018 found that Latinos and African Americans were *more* likely than whites to meet depression criteria.[36] The mixed data may be due to the paucity of research in these community groups, different symptom presentation, or bias among care providers, who may not recognize symptoms as indicative of mental health issues[37]—not because these groups are somehow immune to mental suffering. Those with intersectional identities appear to face even more disparities. For instance, transgender individuals who identify as African American or Black, Hispanic or Latinx, Indigenous, or multiracial are at an increased risk of suicide attempts compared with white transgender individuals.[38]

Most racialized groups face more stigma and shame related to mental illness than white groups. One 2020 review of almost 200,000 participants found that mental illness stigma is higher among ethnic minorities than majorities, and that this gets compounded when stigma overlaps with other social adversity, such as gender discrimination.[39] Another large study found that stigma was associated with lower use of mental health services among Black women of lower socioeconomic backgrounds.[40] As in Katherine's case, some cultural beliefs equate mental illness with weakness that brings shame on the family unit. There may be denial that mental illness even exists or superstitious beliefs about mental illness (such as the belief that demons or evil spirits are the culprit, as I learned about in Lindsay Wong's darkly funny memoir *The Woo-Woo: How I Survived Ice Hockey, Drug Raids, Demons, and My Crazy Chinese Family*).[41]

In addition to cultures having different understandings of mental illness, there are also meaningful care approaches within communities that don't rely on the Western medical model. In a study of Labrador Innu healing approaches to mental distress, the researchers write, "Participants' stories of healing recounted a tragic event that placed them 'under a blanket' for a time, following which they found spiritual strength to extend their hands out to be helped or to recognize resources around them."[42] While Western research has started to address equity disparities in mental health care, it's helpful to remember that healing practices may not be the same from one group to another.

It's also important to be aware of the concept that author and psychotherapist Resmaa Menakem calls "white-body supremacy."[43] Most people are likely familiar with the term "white supremacy," which represents a social system in which white people hold the balance of power. Menakem suggests that white-*body* supremacy is a better way of acknowledging and addressing the trauma that Black and Brown bodies have experienced from this violent system, which can manifest as physical and mental health symptoms. (Menakem argues that white people have been affected by this system as well, and I would encourage white readers to check out his writings and teachings on this topic.)[44]

White-body supremacy also leads to white bodies being held up as the standard against which all other bodies are measured, just as the male body has been held up as the standard against the female body.

In *Unwell Women*, author Elinor Cleghorn writes that throughout Western history, "theories about female neuroses frequently assumed the sufferer was white and affluent, while the plight of working-class women and Black, Asian, and other ethnically diverse women was scarcely, if ever, thought about seriously."[45] Black women and other women of color were thought to be impervious to both mental and physical pain, while white women were considered weak and vulnerable. These beliefs have persisted. A 2016 study found that half of the sampled white medical students and residents endorsed the belief that "Black people's skin is thicker than white people's skin" and rated Black patients' pain as lower.[46]

Stereotypes like these led to what Menakem calls a "strange, contradictory myth" that "it's the job of Black bodies to care for white bodies, soothe them, and protect them—particularly from other Black bodies."[47] Historically, this occurred most often in private homes as Black people served wealthy white families, and in the present day there is a disproportionate representation of Black women (and other women of color) in caregiving roles, as childcare providers and personal support workers or nurses.[48]

In the mental health field, white people are overrepresented in higher-level positions. A 2015 report from the American Psychological Association found that 86 percent of psychologists in the U.S. were white.[49] Meanwhile, Black women and other racialized women are overrepresented in health care in the most hazardous and lowest-wage jobs, such as community or behavioral workers.[50]

Because of culturally constructed ideas about race and pain, there is a myth that racialized women don't suffer as much from mental illness. This phenomenon has been documented in research and shown to intensify Black women's psychological distress. Though this myth is often held up within Black communities, the idea of the strong Black woman has its roots in slavery, and it was used by enslavers to justify slavery.[51] In *The Strong Black Woman: How a Myth Endangers the Physical and Mental Health of Black Women*,

Marita Golden writes, "The Strong Black Woman Syndrome, which requires that Black women perpetually present an image of control and strength, is a response to a combination of daily pressures and systemic racist assaults ... [The syndrome] silences the healthy and necessary expression of pain and vulnerability."[52]

"I WANT TO SET AN EXAMPLE for Black women to not be ashamed to speak about their experiences and their truth," says Tammy Reese, an actress and writer living in Syracuse, New York. Tammy's career began at the age of twelve when she joined the Media Unit, a now defunct New York State youth stage production company. She performed extensively in theater and on television and is an award-winning writer, journalist, director, and producer. Tammy grew up in a middle-class family in what she describes as "the hood" in the Southside neighborhood of Syracuse. Both her parents were well-known in the community, with her father a United States Army veteran and her mother a civil rights and disability activist. "I came from these wholesome, notable 'public figure' parents in our community," she says.

The pressures of her teen years were intensified by a performing schedule that included sixty live stage shows each year and hosting a public access television program. "I lived two lives as a teenager: of trying to get my name out there as a community artist, and then living in the hood and trying to fit in with my friends," she says. Many of her friends were involved in gangs or sold and did drugs. Over the years, the number of people in her life lost to illness or drug and gang violence mounted. Tammy herself fell into drug use, while still maintaining a grueling acting schedule.

Around this time her mother was diagnosed with glaucoma and gradually lost her sight, which meant she and the family had to adjust to a new way of life. Tammy says seeing her mother become depressed by her disability drained her, and she ended up in therapy, wanting to give up on her work as a public figure in order to focus on the needs of her family. It was a dark time, but she also remembers that it united her with her mother's own emotional and physical struggle. They faced depression together.

CULTURALLY COMPETENT CARE

TAMMY'S FIRST EFFORT to reach out for professional help left much to be desired. Her family doctor told her she was simply stressed out, but Tammy knew enough about herself to know that something wasn't right. "When I'd wake up, my back hurt, my neck hurt, my head hurt, and I was feeling nauseous. I didn't want to drive in a car no more . . . and I panicked when I was in the grocery store." She ended up calling a local mental health service center, which was covered under her insurance plan. "They wanted to know: Did I want to do individual services, family services, group counseling?" Tammy said, "I'm going to take all of it."

Tammy's therapist for one-on-one counseling was white, and she remembers initially wanting to talk to someone who looked like her and better understood her lived experience. "It's already hard for Black people to even be vulnerable in a professional therapy session like that," she says. "But she went above my wildest expectations." The therapist regularly checked in with Tammy and showed a level of care that Tammy felt made all the difference for her recovery. "I could really talk to this woman about any- and everything that I was not comfortable talking about with anyone else on the face of the earth—and it was so relieving."

While Tammy's relationship with her therapist was a good one, not everyone has such a positive experience in finding a therapist who is culturally competent. Some therapists assume a standard approach works for all patients, regardless of their identities or experiences. For instance, a Westernized treatment approach tends to be very individualistic, whereas many people come from collectivist cultures, where families and group relationships are much more important. Some therapists or psychiatrists suggest that patients cut ties with problematic family members to set healthy boundaries and pursue a more individualized approach to healing. But such recommendations can run counter to deeply held cultural beliefs about familial obligation, and patients might choose to discontinue treatment when their therapists (though well-intentioned) misunderstand their experience and provide poor advice.[53]

Some patients are speaking out about oppressive practices or ignorant attitudes they've had to deal with in therapy. In one example reported by *Asparagus Magazine*, a patient, who was South Asian, was misgendered and told by the practitioner to try yoga for their mental health, with no understanding that many people from South Asia may already have close ties with yoga as a spiritual and cultural practice (and not as a wellness routine).[54]

Returning to Katherine's story, she highlights how important it was to find a therapist that understood at least one part of her lived experience. "Especially for me, as a fat woman, that's a very specific kind of experience, and . . . my therapist is a fat woman," she says. "So if I talk about stuff, like the assumptions that people make or the comments, she totally understands."

On the other hand, Katherine does wonder if sometimes her therapist doesn't understand her cultural experiences as well. "So sometimes it's like, okay, she can get what it's like to be a fat woman, but when I'm telling her about stuff that comes up because of cultural issues, I can sometimes feel like it's hard to make her understand just how deeply ingrained these things are." When patients receive poor care or experience microaggressions at the hands of their care provider, it can decrease their willingness to adhere to treatment. They are very likely to miss appointments or cancel treatment altogether, and potentially discourage others in their community from seeking treatment as well.[55] Culturally competent providers strive to understand the complex needs of racialized individuals and practice sensitive care for their patients.

Tammy talks about these complex needs, and she laments the fact that Black women's emotions are belittled in our society and our health care system. "We're stereotyped as the 'angry Black woman,'" she says, which becomes part of a vicious cycle. The burden of this stereotype creates a sense of helplessness and despair, and Black women feel that there's no point in trying to get help, because no one cares. These feelings turn into anger, feeding back into the stereotype and ultimately confirming what the woman believes about the health care system and its inability to provide her with proper support. Tammy says that many Black women try to overcompensate to deal with stereotypes. "We have to overwork ourselves to prove to society that we're not just some ghetto Black woman; we are educated, we are smart, we are talented, we are strong." It is an exhausting situation to be in, and Tammy sees many Black women who feel they have to mask their pain.

Tammy is working hard to change the narrative in her community through her work as a public figure. "I want . . . to appeal to my Black women counterparts that we have to stop saying that 'Oh, therapy is a white people thing,'" she says. "I don't care what color you are, how much money you've got, where you went to school. Listen, everybody can be affected by mental illness."

I ask Tammy what needs to change for American women, and Black American women in particular, when it comes to mental health services. "First, I would say the key is to listen," she says. Even though the doctor didn't outright say "Oh, you'll be all right" and pat her on the back, Tammy felt that this is what they were implying: that she was just stressed out and needed to rest. It felt like a glib response to a serious situation. "I know they went to school for all these years . . . but you can't go to school to learn how someone else feels," she says. On the flip side, Tammy knows that patients aren't doctors. "So it's like a mutual conversation of building an understanding that this person is telling you what's going on, and this isn't normal."

The reality is not every patient will be matched with a care provider who meets their specific cultural background. Strategies are needed to increase the diversity of psychologists and psychiatrists, but culturally competent care is still possible between two people of different backgrounds. It takes training and education, active listening, and an acceptance that the providers might not have all the answers.

The concept of listening to a patient, seeing the situation from their point of view, and adopting an attitude of humility is not something that all mental health care providers do well, Wieman tells me. This kind of approach to care requires clinicians to accept that they will never fully understand their patients; many instead push back against their feelings of uncertainty and double down on provider-led decision-making. This sometimes means that patients do not fully understand what is happening to them or do not accept the decision that is being made. If the patient is well resourced, they may seek care elsewhere to get their needs met. But for many women facing the barriers we've covered in this chapter, they may abandon care altogether.

MENTAL HEALTH FOR ALL PEOPLE

"THERE COMES A POINT where we need to stop just pulling people out of the river. We need to go upstream and find out why they're falling in."

This powerful quote has been attributed to Desmond Tutu, but I couldn't find any evidence he ever wrote or said these words. However, I did find a 1975 paper (since republished) about "upstream factors" to public health. In it, John McKinlay lays out his case for tackling "manufacturers of illness," which he defines as the economic forces that are responsible for much of the illness and death we face in our society.[56] Health care workers are receiving people downstream, when symptoms and outcomes are at their worst. Upstream, economic and cultural forces continue to shove people into the water, and this is where much of our effort should be focused.

I suspect that most care providers working in the Western mental health system acknowledge that these upstream factors need to be addressed, but figuring out how is up for debate. The capitalist approach is to frame mental health as a supply-demand problem. "Demand" is the number of people who self-report feeling mental distress, or the number of people who have received *DSM* diagnoses in a specific area or country. But "demand" isn't necessarily the same as "want" or "need," and we can see from the survey data I shared earlier in this chapter that unmet needs vary. Depending on their social and economic circumstances, some women may not feel comfortable expressing their needs or may face barriers if they do. On the supply side, throwing more care providers or money at the problem (what is referred to as the "spray and pray" method) has not led to an improved system when the *quality* of those services is lacking.

An alternative approach is to fund a mental health system that promotes human rights.[57] Proponents of this model suggest that the overmedicalization of mental health has led to coercion (for example, people being forcibly admitted to institutions and being denied their legal capacity), denial of life in the community, and pathologizing normal human experiences. These proponents are not arguing that we do away with the medical model of health care; instead, the idea is for people to have the right to choose a range of services, from community- or family-based supports to medication and psychiatric care.

If we were to lead with this model, increased funding for mental health would be aligned with the United Nations Convention on the Rights of Persons with Disabilities (CRPD), which includes people with psychosocial disabilities (i.e., mental disorders). The CRPD has been ratified by 181 countries to protect and promote the right to health through a lens of dignity, autonomy, and life in the community.

In high-income countries, 43 percent of all spending for mental health is for hospital-related services and costs; in low-income countries, this figure is a whopping 80 percent.[58] Even when funding is channeled to the community, the services tend to be medical—for example, the primary care delivery of antidepressant or depressant medication.

A human rights perspective looks more closely at the nature of the services being funded, shifting from a disease model toward a system that funds nonclinical services (such as the community mental health centers in the U.S.), peer support, and building a person's legal capacity so that they can participate fully in decision-making and do not feel coerced into certain treatments.

I was excited to learn more about this model, but I also felt wary—could a system that focuses on human rights actually lead to improved access to care and a more supportive system for women? To explore an on-the-ground example that uses a human rights approach, I turned my attention to Pune, India, where the experience of a Tamil woman named Bapu became the catalyst for an entirely different kind of mental health care.

Bapu was born under colonial rule in India at a time when psychiatric asylums were the only option for people suffering from mental disorders.[59] According to family members, Bapu "went mad" after the birth of her two children and began having religious visions and hearing voices. She gave up the culturally prescribed role of mother and housemaker to live a religious life, dressing in monk's clothing and following strict spiritual practices. Bapu was eventually diagnosed with schizophrenia in the 1960s, and she endured years of forced confinement in psychiatric institutions, invasive treatments, and medications that left her with debilitating side effects. After escaping these institutions and having multiple run-ins with police, Bapu became homeless and disappeared for many years. She was eventually found by one of her children who "carried her small, frail body in his arms and brought her back home." She died soon after, in 1996.[60]

There are striking similarities to my grandmother's story here, though, of course, Bapu suffered in a different decade and in a different country. Yet the notion of coercive care holds true for Kit's experience. My grandmother never chose medication or institutionalization (in fact, there were times she outright refused them), but those were the only options that our family could access, and we were led to believe that this was best for her. Furthermore, as primary caregivers, our family had no one else to fall back on as we navigated the chaotic situation. Beyond immediate family members and psychiatrists, there was no circle of care that could help address the layers of challenges my grandmother faced, including trauma, emotional abuse, and financial pressures.

In honor of Bapu and the horrific treatment she faced, one of her children formed a charitable trust in her name. One of their programs, called Seher, aims to fulfill the standards of the CRPD with zero coercion. Rather than classifying mental disorders into a binary of "severe" versus "common," Seher understands mental health as a spectrum, ranging from low-support to high-support needs and consisting of many different aspects, including stressors of daily living and psychological distress. Defining its main outcome as social inclusion rather than treatment, the program assesses a person's needs (rather than making a DSM diagnosis based on symptoms), examines what they're missing in terms of social, economic, family, and therapeutic supports, and offers a full range of community-based services to meet those needs.

Seher builds what it calls a "Circle of Care"—a supportive network of family, friends, or neighbors—as well as using self-care tools (for example, breathing exercises) and social justice interventions (for example, addressing issues of violence). The program also offers nutrition assistance and health care and organizes peer groups, informal counseling, and arts-based programs. Psychiatric solutions are an option, but Seher also supports individuals who want to withdraw from psychiatric drugs.[61]

In a chapter of *Mental Health, Legal Capacity, and Human Rights*, I read about the case of Meera, a pseudonym for a thirty-two-year-old woman living with her mother and brother. Meera was dealing with multiple disabilities, including epilepsy, and her greatest need was an epilepsy diagnosis and treatment. Seher provided Meera and her family with food when supplies were low. The team arranged to get Meera a monthly disability pension, offered her training and support so that she could live independently, and provided basic counseling services and an arts program. And the team went even further: they worked on neighborhood dialogue and education to reduce the violence and bullying she'd been experiencing in the community. It seems like a dizzying array of supports, but without those basic needs being met, I suspect Meera's path to healing would not have been as successful.[62]

The Bapu Trust is not the only example of innovative and socially focused mental health care. Here in Canada, I've been following the social prescribing movement—an approach that seems very similar to what I describe above. Social prescribing brings nonclinical health care services closer together in the community and directly addresses issues like housing, financial insecurity, loneliness, and social isolation. While it's not specific to mental health, its main goal is to address the underlying causes of an illness as opposed to treating symptoms. Just like Seher, a program of social prescribing links people with local low-cost services that are easy to access—anything from an arts program to assistance with affordable housing. Studies that evaluate social prescribing have found that it can reduce visits to family doctors or the emergency room, improve psychological well-being, and increase a person's perceived quality of life.[63]

One of the biggest barriers to implementing social prescribing more widely for mental health issues is that someone needs to do the work of linking a person with services. Research has shown that many family doctors lack training and time to address social issues and mental illness. (And here in Canada, millions of people are living without a family doctor, which means they're relying on walk-in services and emergency rooms for basic medical care.) Link workers, who liaise with doctors and their patients on the ground in communities, may be able to fill the gap between primary care and community support.[64]

Another barrier is philosophical—how we think and talk about mental illness and mental health. As I've argued, we have an overwhelming tendency to pathologize women's emotional and physical symptoms, seeing mental illness as an individual mind-body problem. For the wider system of care to shift from a medical model to a social model, we need to reimagine what "mentally ill" truly means.

5

THE CULTURAL CONSTRUCTION OF MENTAL ILLNESS

In undergrad, I used to poke fun at psychology—a soft science. It was about the brain and cognition, yes, but it was also about mood—feelings and emotions created by the human mind. Those feelings and emotions seemed useless to me if I couldn't locate them in data, if I couldn't see how the nervous system worked by taking it apart.

YAA GYASI'

THE OCCULT SHOP was once located in a squat brownstone building behind my apartment, in the bustling Wychwood neighborhood of Toronto. The store carried a range of occult and pagan supplies, with bins of crystals, sticks of incense, and rows of jarred herbs lining the walls. It also provided tarot readings, and a good friend decided a reading was exactly what I needed for my twenty-fifth birthday. I think she wanted to bust me out of my frequent doldrums—loosen me from the undercurrent of depression in my early adult life. Maybe a hopeful picture of my future success was the inspiration I needed.

I stepped into the back of the shop through a black curtain, terrified I would be met with an older woman sporting a turban and massaging a crystal ball. Instead, I was greeted by a young guy wearing jeans and a T-shirt. He sat down behind a small desk and welcomed me to take the seat in front of him. I perched awkwardly on the edge of the chair, still looking around for signs of the crystal ball, but instead saw a stack of thick tarot cards lying on the desk beside him.

"What brings you in today?" he asked in a friendly voice.

My reply was something along the lines of "My friend dragged me here, so I'm not really sure." Instead of picking up the cards, he observed me, noting the energy that he was seeing.

"I see so much going on around your head," he said. "It's like a busy highway up there! But below your neck—there's nothing."

"Great," I thought. "I'm dead inside."

"There's a big disconnect between your mind and your body," he continued. "Have you ever tried sitting quietly and breathing deeply into your belly?"

While I had dabbled in the occasional yoga class after my first breakdown, deep breathing was not something I regularly did. It almost always triggered a sense of panic. A full breath acted like a fan for thousands of spastic butterflies roaming my abdomen. My throat would constrict, and soon I would have to abandon the whole process, terrified I might trigger a full-blown panic attack. I found it easier to ignore my body entirely, hoping that I could get through each miserable day by willpower alone.

WHERE DOES IT HURT?

WHEN I FIRST GOT SICK, it was difficult to discern whether I was struggling with a physical illness or something that existed only in the mind. Did I need to see a gastroenterologist or a psychiatrist? In the beginning, my doctors went the physical route, and I submitted to scopes, scans, and tests to ascertain if my stomach troubles stemmed from a disease of the body. When all tests came back clear, my symptoms then became a functional problem; there was no scientific explanation for why I was experiencing panic attacks, nausea, and irritable bowel. The search for an identifiable disease ended. My doctors instead believed that my symptoms were psychosomatic—that my mind was creating a pattern of physical illness that others who have a "true" disease exhibit. I was not alone; it's been estimated that 30 to 40 percent of patients experience mental distress in the form of physical symptoms.[2]

By that time, my mental problems were being treated by a psychologist and a psychiatrist, who led me to believe that there was a brain-based explanation for my symptoms. It's likely that no brain scan or genetic test could have ever revealed the source of my distress, yet the hunt for a treatment to help me often rested on the premise of a biological basis for my problems.

There continues to be tension in the mental health field over how to define the "mind." Is it a physical thing that we have yet to fully measure and quantify using the handy tools of scientific inquiry? Does it exist within the body, and does it depend on the functioning of the brain? Freud's understanding (although this came later in his career) was that depression and anxiety were psychological in nature, arising from some deep wound of the mind or soul.

In Western culture, the idea of the mind-body is often reduced to a brain-body connection, with a corresponding belief that our thoughts, emotions, feelings, perceptions, and experiences all arise physically in the shape of neurological structure and nervous system processes. Current popular and scientific thinking define the "mind" as the physical brain, with the nervous system being responsible for the functions of our body. Our system of care focuses largely on the premise that all mental illness will one day be attributable to a problem in the brain.[3]

Allan H. Ropper and Brian David Burrell, whom you may recall from Chapter 1, write about the swinging pendulum between mind and brain in their book *How the Brain Lost Its Mind: Sex, Hysteria, and the Riddle of Mental Illness.* When Ropper first started practicing medicine in the late 1970s, he noticed that patients suffering from mental illness wanted to understand what events in their lives had led to their distress, and physicians were happy to oblige them. The longer he practiced, the more he noticed a trend in the medical community that implicated brain processes in mental disorders. Patients, in turn, sought a biological explanation for their problems.[4] Which isn't necessarily a bad thing—we all want to know why or how we found ourselves in such a bad place, and a physical explanation can be soothing.

However, when we believe that all of our problems arise from disordered brain processes, we may perceive psychological interventions as being less helpful in our recovery.[5] In one study of 279 patients at a psychiatric hospital, researchers found that a belief in the chemical imbalance theory of mental illness led to lowered expectations of psychological treatment efficacy.[6] It's possible that when we have greater pessimism about the functioning of our brain, we feel we have little power over our situation and less ability to foster change.[7] In my own experience, I assumed my grandmother had passed along her poorly functioning brain chemicals to me and that I was (and always would be) "mentally ill."

The great leaps forward we have made in brain imaging, gene mapping, and biochemistry may one day reveal to us unique biological causes for mental illness, but without considering a person's lived experience (which I would include in a definition of the "mind"), we might never understand the psychological side of mental illness. Ropper and Burrell write that the same can be said in reverse, in that "no amount of parsing of the contents of mental illness can explain much about the corresponding brain illness."[8] By "contents," they are referring to our thoughts and experiences, or what they believe makes up the mind. They argue that the connection between the brain and the mind is not one-way or predictable, cautioning that the brain is "not a Rube Goldberg device in which sensory experience goes in one end and stimulates a pinball firing of neurons [nerve cells], and thoughts come out the other end."[9] In other words, it's not cause and effect but a chaotic mess of two-way interactions between all the moving biopsychosocial parts—what makes you a whole person.

Just as there is confusion over the source of mental illness—whether it resides in the mind or the brain—there is disagreement over how we define mental disorders and discern between "normal" and "disordered" thinking, emotions, and behaviors.

LABELS: THE GOOD,
THE BAD, AND THE MOODY

"WHO GETS TO DEFINE NORMAL?"

I posed this question one day while I sat in a circle facing eight young women at a peer support group for people struggling with eating disorders. As the facilitator, I was open and honest about my past struggles with food, weight, and depression. No one was looking to me as the expert, but I was far enough along in my recovery that I could lead the group with open-ended questions and gentle activities to bring us to a deeper understanding of our own path to healing.

The answers came fast:

"My mother."

"My doctor."

"My psychiatrist."

"My partner."

"Society."

Not a single one of them said "Me."

As girls and women, we do not get the luxury of defining what is normal when it comes to our thoughts, emotions, and behavior. "I like to use glasses as a metaphor here," says Lindsey Boes, a marriage and family therapist in private practice. "It's the lens through which we see everything—even our own reflection in the mirror is influenced by these lenses of social norms and dominant cultural practices. Things like toxic individuality and tenets of white supremacy, like perfectionism, defensiveness, and fear of open conflict; all of these different power structures that we soak up influence the way we make sense of ourselves and the stories that we tell."

Instead of learning how to make sense of our own stories in relation to the world around us, women have our symptoms and experiences pathologized as abnormal, and we are diagnosed with a disease—what might be called "a statistical deviation from normal functioning."[10] In the mental health and scientific world, we have defined what is normal in gendered ways. "Women are depressed and women are anxious and women have trauma," says Boes. "It's just a 'woman thing,' and then people socialized as men aren't getting access to explore all of their emotions, and so those emotions just come out as anger—and we don't diagnose men for being angry, because there isn't a diagnosis for this."

Using Boes's glasses metaphor again, one way to look at psychological disorder or dysfunction is through the lens of social constructivism, a philosophy that proposes that society determines what is considered normal and that anything that deviates from that norm becomes medicalized.[11] Perhaps one of the most radical proponents of this view was Thomas Szasz, who argued that mental illness is a myth, because there is no discernible problem with the body or brain. He instead felt that psychiatric diagnoses are aimed at repressing socially undesirable behavior.[12]

Those of us who have faced severe mental illness would likely counter that our suffering or the suffering of our loved ones is indeed real and has significant consequences for our health and ability to function within society. Kristen Lindquist, whom you met in Chapter 2, tells me that while it's helpful to understand how the concept of mental illness and its symptoms have been culturally defined, we still don't want to ignore biological experiences.

"As a neuroscientist, I am certainly not trying to suggest that there isn't some biology that is contributing to people's experiences," she says. "If you focus on the conceptual knowledge side of things, like where did the categories come from and what is their specific meaning, and what sort of baggage do they come with—a lot of that is socialized."

Since the early understandings of mental illness as a medical problem, diagnostic categories of what is normal and what is disease have been constantly evolving. It was psychiatrist Emil Kraepelin who penned the popular tome *Compendium der Psychiatrie*, first published in the late nineteenth century and revised as a three-thousand-page, four-volume textbook in 1915.[13] He used his experimental observations (which also became the basis for contemporary pharmacological research) to create categories of mental diagnoses, based in his belief that mental illness was a biological disease of the brain. Prior to the DSM, Kraepelin's classification system guided clinical psychiatry for much of the early twentieth century.

In his book *A Cure for Darkness*, writer and depression sufferer Alex Riley gives a fascinating account of Kraepelin's life and work, noting that "Kraepelin was his own worst critic" and readily admitted to the shortcomings of his classification system. Riley quotes from the psychiatrist's famous *Lectures on Clinical Psychiatry*, in which Kraepelin says, "We are still so far removed from a real knowledge of the causes, phenomena, course, and termination of the individual forms [of mental disorder] that we cannot yet dream of a surely established edifice of knowledge at all."[14] In other words, he didn't feel sure there was any solid evidence for the categories he'd created.

The field has come a long way since 1915. We know so much more about mental illness now than we did back then, and the *DSM* has been revised five times by groups of clinical experts. However, skepticism remains within the mental health field over whether the *DSM* is an accurate classification of mental illness. One of the main criticisms of the latest edition (*DSM-5* in 2013) is that the thresholds to diagnose an individual with a mental disorder have been lowered for most classifications, meaning more people are receiving diagnoses. This comes with a risk of pathologizing normal human emotions. For example, the *DSM-5* now allows for an individual's grief after a loss to be diagnosed as major depression without any time limits. (A previous version cited two months after the loss as the threshold, which was arbitrary and not grounded in evidence.) Critics would contend that grief is a normal—albeit very challenging—emotional process that shouldn't be pathologized.[15]

Over the years, I've had niggling doubts about my own diagnoses—all five of them. I received each diagnosis from a different practitioner over a span of fifteen years; with each new label, I assumed that my mental illness had simply changed tack. It started as panic, became generalized anxiety, morphed into an eating disorder, was revised as cyclothymia—a condition that shares many similarities with bipolar disorder—and finally culminated in a bout of postpartum mood disorder.

Digging deeper, I came to realize that the tools we use to diagnose mental illness rely heavily on a clinician's subjective (and often biased) beliefs about an individual rather than on evidence-based and scientific measures. Diagnosing physical illness is a much more objective task, with biomarkers that tell us whether our insulin or cholesterol is too high, scans that can spot burst appendices or dreaded tumors, and countless diagnostic tools to guide doctors in their treatment decisions.

Racial, gender, and other biases in the classification of mental disorders also mean that certain populations are diagnosed at much higher rates than others. In the book *(Mis)diagnosed: How Bias Distorts Our Perception of Mental Health*, social worker Jonathan Foiles explains that mental diseases are unlike any other bodily illness in that they are disorders of function instead of an abnormality in the role or structure of an organ. "That is, they are diagnosed based upon what one *does*," he writes.[16]

Foiles examines several different biases and how they distort our perception of mental health. Black men are more likely to be diagnosed with schizophrenia compared to other racialized or white men; white children have much higher rates of ADHD (and receive better support and care) than racialized children; the LGBTQ+ community has long been targeted by DSM diagnoses (homosexuality as a mental disorder was only removed from the DSM in 1973 and was replaced with "sexual orientation disturbance," which pathologized people who felt distress over their sexuality); and there is bias against people with intellectual disabilities, which are diagnosed partly through IQ scores—a scale with a decidedly questionable scientific basis.[17]

Foiles writes that "psychology does not exist above and beyond our prejudices, no matter how much it aspires to scientific objectivity. It has too often started not with a concern for the mental health of others but rather our own discomfort, and mental illness becomes the label we use to classify that discomfort by reassuring ourselves that 'they' are the problem."[18]

One mental disorder label is used far more frequently for women than it is for men, in order to categorize a pattern of behavior that society finds altogether displeasing.

LIVING ON THE PERIPHERY

FREUD BELIEVED THAT society was built upon our suppression of our basic (read: sexual) instincts. The rational or "thinking" brain stamped out that hardwired reptilian brain to repress our animalistic desires. This is what's called the "triune brain" theory, which proposed that humans possess an ancient lizard brain topped with an emotional mammalian brain and finished off with a human rational brain. This theory has since been debunked, and neuroscientific research has proven that our brains never evolved that way.[19]

Because of all this hard work we were supposedly doing to suppress our raging sexuality, Freud believed two nervous disorders could result. The first he called neurosis, the run-of-the-mill depression and anxiety so many of us experience throughout our lives. The other he called psychoneurosis, which he saw as being part of the body and not solely located in the unconscious mind—this is where he dumped all the unfortunate hysterical women.[20]

The women who fell somewhere in the middle between neurotic and psychotic were placed on the periphery; they were "borderline." While neurotics and psychotics were easy to diagnose based on their neat categorical symptoms, Foiles argues that those with "borderline" (what became known as borderline personality disorder, or BPD) "lack[ed] such stability, a sense of a continuity of character from one moment to the next."[21]

CHARLEY KNOWS EXACTLY what it's like to live in liminal spaces, as a person with lived experience in the mental health care system and as a care provider treating people with mental illness. She began having mental health difficulties in her early teen years and struggled with low mood and self-harm throughout high school. At sixteen, she developed an eating disorder and spent half a year living as an inpatient on a psychiatric unit in the U.K., as there were few services to support her in her small rural community. Her personal experience piqued her interest in working in the field of mental health, and she set out to study psychology, a practice she says spoke to her general approach to mental health challenges. But despite the treatments she received for her own illness and the sense of purpose she discovered on her path to becoming a psychologist, she continued to struggle with her mental health. "I hadn't really addressed anything properly from my past," she says.

Post-university, Charley found herself in the same place as so many other young people after graduation: no sense of direction, no money, and struggling to find a decent job. "Things just started to get worse and worse, and I was on a really long waiting list for NHS treatment," says Charley. "And during that time, I made an attempt to end my life."

The care she received at the hospital after her suicide attempt involved a twenty-minute assessment with a liaison psychiatrist, who deemed Charley safe to go home. After this, she waited five weeks for an appointment with a psychiatric nurse at a community mental health center. The nurse spent forty-five minutes with Charley, taking a health history and chatting about her current struggles. She remembers getting called back into the room with the nurse and a psychiatrist and being told that she was diagnosed with BPD. "I burst into tears because I worked as an assistant psychologist at that time, and I knew what that label meant ... I knew full well the stigma," says Charley. "I'd heard nurses say at work, 'Ignore them, they're PD,' or 'They're just attention-seeking, they're PD.'" For Charley, the diagnosis was devastating because she had witnessed firsthand how BPD patients were treated in the system. She asked the psychiatrist not to put the diagnosis in her record, knowing that the label would follow her throughout her life and career. She worried no one would ever take her seriously again.

"They refused to listen to me, and it went down on my history," she says. "That was a label given to me by somebody who had met me once for the first time on that day; they really didn't know that much about me."

In the psychiatric tome of diagnostic labels, BPD continues to carry a strong Freudian interpretation. According to Foiles, people with BPD are described culturally as "manipulative, needy, seductive, and fearful of rejection"—in essence, they are drama.[22] The crazy ex-girlfriend. The bridezilla. The psycho bitch. We could replace those terms with ghosts from years past, such as "hysteric" and "witch," and conclude that a tiger can never change its stripes. Hysteria lives on in many forms, but BPD may be one of the most significant; the *DSM-IV* stated that BPD is diagnosed predominantly (about 75 percent) in women.[23] Since the publication of the *DSM-5* in 2013, one large survey suggested that men are also suffering from BPD but that there may be sex or gender differences in how the disorder manifests; women appear to have greater mental and physical disabilities associated with the illness.[24] Bias in the diagnosis of BPD has also been observed for LGBTQ+ patients, which may mean that clinicians are predisposed to see BPD traits in this group.[25]

What almost all of those who are diagnosed with BPD seem to have in common is a history of trauma. As Charley points out, people with BPD are behaving in ways that at one point were important survival strategies, and they were *effective*. "When I was a twelve- or thirteen-year-old being groomed by an adult man and I didn't have any friends and nobody to talk to, I suppose self-harm was an effective strategy for me at that point," she says. "Because it helped me cope."

In an article for *The Conversation*, Australian psychiatrist Jayashri Kulkarni and researcher Patrick Walker argue that BPD is in fact a complex response to trauma rather than a personality disorder. "The similarities between complex PTSD and BPD are numerous. Patients with both conditions have difficulty regulating their emotions; they experience persistent feelings of emptiness, shame, and guilt; and they have a significantly elevated risk of suicide," they write.[26]

Another interesting dimension of BPD is that it appears to have significant overlap with autism spectrum conditions, which could partially explain why girls and women are diagnosed with autism at a much lower rate than boys and men—they're likely receiving other mental health labels instead.[27]

The BPD label is such a significant problem for women because it translates as a personality flaw. Patients often believe that the disorder is their own fault, which leads to a sense of worthlessness and a lack of agency. And as Charley witnessed in her work, care providers often view these patients as manipulative and attention-seeking, whereas someone with PTSD and complex trauma is usually viewed in a sympathetic light, because we understand that something very bad must have occurred for the person to have reached such a level of distress.

Some argue that labels for mental illness benefit patients with the validation that comes with a diagnosis. A person can feel a sense of relief that someone has finally named their pain and that they share this pain with many other people all around the world. But the benefits of a diagnostic label are sometimes outweighed by stigma and feelings of shame or brokenness, particularly for a condition like BPD.

"When I first read about BPD, it did resonate," says Charley. "I thought, 'Oh my God, that's me.' I'm terrified of being abandoned, I've had a history of eating disorders . . . and self-harm." She describes seeing the symptoms and thinking "Tick, tick, tick" as each box was checked. Nonetheless, Charley points out that a person only needs five symptoms out of a possible nine for a diagnosis of BPD. Many of these symptoms overlap with other mental disorders: suicidal behavior, mood swings, constant feelings of worthlessness or sadness, and loss of contact with reality. "So people can present completely differently and still get the same label put on them, which shows really that it's not a scientific or actual syndrome," says Charley. "It does just feel like a catchall for the more difficult people."

IF WE COMPARE the listed symptoms for most major mental disorders, we see that many symptoms overlap, creating a complicated network of human suffering. A network map of mental disorders, created by researchers at the University of Amsterdam, looks like a beautiful night sky, with stars shooting off in every direction.[28] But when I reflect on the diagram with my diagnoses in mind, it becomes difficult to understand how the DSM categories hold any real significance. There is no clear delineation between the many labels applied to folks struggling with similar symptoms.

A network theory of common mental disorders argues that problems may arise from an interaction *between* symptoms, because there's often nothing we can point to as "diseased" in the body.[29] For example, maybe I'm feeling stressed over a big project at work, so I don't sleep well one night. I'm very tired the following day, which fuels further worries about whether I'll be able to sleep the following night, and soon this pattern progresses to insomnia. As my symptoms continue to intermingle, my doctor uses a screening tool that identifies several symptoms of an anxiety disorder (fatigue, difficulty controlling worry, and trouble sleeping), and I am given a diagnosis.

The traditional explanation for this anxiety disorder is that there's some underlying factor that's *caused* my distress; the network theory proposes instead that mental disorders involve a feedback-loop process of various symptoms all interacting with each other. It's an interesting theory, because it means that we could chart an individual's symptom network and target one of the central symptoms to see how it affects the others. In the case of my worry → insomnia → anxiety example (which has indeed happened to me many times over the years), my doctor might target sleep through healthy sleep habits, mindfulness practices, and sleep medication, if needed. Once I'm sleeping better, my other symptoms might resolve.

I want to be clear here that I'm not arguing we throw the *DSM* in the trash (although there are other books on this topic that would suggest that). Depending on the country in which you live, doing away with mental health diagnoses in the current political and legal systems would ultimately be harmful to many people. In my own country, the Mental Health Commission of Canada estimates that 30 percent of disability claims can be attributed to mental health issues, with an economic cost exceeding fifty billion dollars annually.[30] A diagnosis is required to access disability benefits, and even with one, some people struggle to get their claims approved.[31] In the U.S., diagnoses are a prerequisite to accessing insurance coverage for mental health services.

"In the U.K., you don't need a diagnosis for treatment services, which helps a lot," says Charley. "It's kind of irrelevant what medical diagnosis a patient has. When the person sits down and starts talking to you, you work with the person that's there." Previous diagnoses may help to inform the psychologist's understanding of an individual's past, but Charley feels that what's more important is to focus on the individual and their current challenges. Now that she has graduated as a qualified clinical psychologist, Charley's dedication to listening to the patient's narrative and providing person-centered care is top of mind.

In many ways, Charley feels that she's come far from the chaotic days of her BPD diagnosis. A therapist she saw privately helped her connect the dots between painful childhood experiences and the distress she was feeling in adulthood. Charley describes how this therapy changed her, saying, "I hold my therapist with me and the stuff that she taught me. I have that compassionate voice inside me...and an awareness of things that I didn't have before."

THE BIOPSYCHOSOCIAL MODEL

SO FAR IN THIS CHAPTER, I've discussed the lack of scientific consensus over where mental illness lives (in the brain, the body, or the mind) and how it gets defined. One man who saw the problems with the mental health system took it upon himself to develop a new theory that he hoped would revamp care for people living with mental illness.

The biopsychosocial model (BPSM), introduced by George Engel in the late 1970s, was supposed to be the answer to the problem with biological psychiatry, which favored drugs over psychosocial approaches to mental health. Biological psychiatry began to take hold in the early twentieth century (with Freud an early proponent before defecting to the dark side of the mind), and it really gained traction after modern antipsychotic and antidepressant drugs were introduced midcentury. The research for these drugs also led to the development of the chemical imbalance theory for mental disorders, linking lowered serotonin to depression.[32]

Engel argued that the biomedical model left no room for the consideration of social, psychological, and environmental aspects of illness. The BPSM was seen both as a game changer for patients in a system that wasn't working very well and as a guide for health care providers seeking ways to do right by people with mental illness.[33] His article introducing BPSM had a big impact on the Western scientific community and has been cited over nineteen thousand times since it was first published.[34]

There was just one key issue with the BPSM: it was widely praised but never really adopted in practice.[35] It's been more than forty years since the introduction of this approach, and the dominant model of disease and treatment remains biomedical. As psychologist Sanah Ahsan writes in *The Guardian*, "In efforts to destigmatise mental distress, 'mental illness' is framed as an 'illness like any other'—rooted in supposedly flawed brain chemistry." Yet, Ahsan argues, the "broken brain" explanation merely increases stigma and disempowerment and distracts us from the social causes of distress.[36]

We aren't practicing true holism (the understanding of the mind-body as singular and interconnected) when we reduce our lived experience to basic biology. When health care providers told me my brain was dysfunctional and that my problem was a chemical imbalance, I had no wider lens through which to view my illness. If I were to argue that women's mental illness is solely biological—perhaps due to genes, chemical imbalances, or hormonal fluctuations—I'd be reducing women to the function of their bodies and once again subscribing to a centuries-old belief that women are in some way broken. Where our uterus, our ovaries, or our minds were once the problem, now it is our brains.

I do understand that for some women, the biological explanation is likely (or at least partially) an accurate one. For people like my grandmother and Patricia, whom you met in Chapter 3, hormonal triggers are a major contributing factor to mental illness. The "mental illness is biological" belief can also be comforting because it helps to elevate mental illness to the status of other physical illnesses, like diabetes or cancer, and makes it more acceptable. Still, I worry that it gives society a get-out-of-jail-free card, where instead of recognizing the complex effects of sexual harassment and abuse, racism, poverty, gender inequality, and trauma, we tell women it's their brains that are the real problem.

Mental illness needs a refresh, in the mind-body philosophies we use to define it and talk about it, as well as in our understanding of how it unfolds in our individual lives and our society. This would help us to address the biases that exist in our perception of women's and girls' mental health and begin to peel back the layers of social influence in emotional distress. Furthermore, I think it would expose two big elephants in the room, or the two systems of oppression that feed off each other to keep women sick and tired: patriarchy and capitalism.

6

THE PROBLEMS
WITH PATRIARCHY

I am not free while any woman is unfree, even when
her shackles are very different from my own.

AUDRE LORDE¹

IN A *FORBES* PIECE recognizing the five-year anniversary
of the viral #MeToo movement, Holly Corbett writes, "At
the root of sexual harassment is power; who has it and
who doesn't. It isn't a single issue, but is deeply intertwined
not only with gender inequities, but also with racial, class,
socioeconomic, and other inequities."² #MeToo's founder
Tarana Burke maintains that the movement's purpose is to
support marginalized people in marginalized communities—not because white women's stories are less important,
but because the experiences of women of color, and of queer
and trans folks, often remain invisible and survivors do not
receive the support they need.³ There are disparities when
it comes to the women who are listened to, believed, and
offered mental health care following sexual harassment.

When I discuss patriarchy in this chapter, I am referring to all the issues converging in this imbalanced system of power that I believe deeply affect women's mental health.

The message girls and young women receive growing up is like a broken record: *not safe, not safe, not safe*. But more than that, they feel unsafe *and* lack the power to change it. Constant vigilance becomes part of a girl's defense mechanism, and many women spend their lives adjusting their own behavior to cope with threats to their safety. The research I've done for this book suggests that when girls and young women lack social safety, their bodies and sense of self can be harmed in measurable and long-lasting ways.

A CONSTANT THREAT

STATISTICS ABOUT SEX- AND GENDER-BASED violence against girls and women are terrifying. As a mother of two girls, I worry constantly about their safety in this world, and I don't think my worries are unfounded. Statistics Canada reports that 30 percent of women aged fifteen and older have been sexually assaulted outside an intimate partner relationship at least once.[4] Globally, one-third of women who have ever been partnered in a relationship experience intimate partner violence.[5] Women living at the intersection of oppressed identities of gender, race, and sexuality (for example, Black LGBTQ+ individuals) may have an elevated risk for sexual violence.[6] In my country, over one thousand Indigenous girls and women were murdered between 1980 and 2012, and that number is likely fourfold greater when taking into account those who have gone missing or whose deaths were misattributed to suicide or accident.[7]

Girls are experiencing violence, sexual assault, or harassment at very young ages, and research has shown that girls who reach puberty earlier than their peers are exposed to more sexual harassment.[8] In a large study that tracked close to eight thousand women over fourteen years, it was found that earlier onset of menstruation was associated with an elevated risk for long-term mental health challenges, which could relate to early exposure to sex- and gender-based violence.[9]

Even when early puberty is not a risk factor, there is anecdotal evidence that girls receive unwanted sexual attention and experience sexual violence throughout adolescence and early adulthood to a much greater extent than boys do. The U.K. website Everyone's Invited was founded as a space for survivors to share their stories anonymously, and since 2020, they have received fifty thousand accounts of sexual violence. These stories are posted publicly, but a big trigger warning if you decide to visit the website—they can be distressing to read. Girls and young women of all ages document stories of violent rape, unwanted touching, street harassment, online sexual abuse, and sexual coercion.[10] There are undoubtedly stories from boys and young men, who also experience harassment and violence, but the reality is that most sexual violence is perpetrated by boys and men against girls and women. In response, the government Office for Standards in Education, Children's Services, and Skills published a report on sexual harassment and online sexual abuse for children and young people in U.K. schools. The report found that nine out of ten girls had received unsolicited sexual images online and had been subject to sexist name-calling.[11]

What does this constant threat of sexual violence do to a young developing girl? The most evident outcome that's backed by research is poorer mental health, including anxiety and depressive symptoms.[12] Women are two to three times as likely to develop PTSD compared to men, with a lifetime prevalence of 10 to 12 percent in women and 5 to 6 percent in men.[13] Girls and women who don't meet diagnostic criteria for PTSD may still be experiencing a stress response that looks very much the same.

Helen Wilson, a clinical psychologist and clinical professor of psychiatry and behavioral sciences at Stanford University, has been studying the effects of trauma across the life span and the relationship between childhood trauma and health risk behavior (for example, engaging in sexually risky behavior) in adolescence and adulthood. In a specific population of Black women, Wilson wanted to know whether other forms of stress and trauma, like microaggression and racism, mattered when it came to outcomes related to "criterion A traumas," such as physical and sexual assault. "And we found that it does seem to matter," she says.

More pervasive, ongoing, repetitive kinds of stressors may not rise to the level of a physical threat. However, "at a very basic level, it doesn't matter whether we're being physically attacked or if it's a more emotional stressor," she says. The brain-body response is very similar.

Wilson tells me that our body's "default" is not a chilled-out state. It's actually a stress response state from the sympathetic nervous system, which helps ensure our survival. It's theorized that the job of the vagus nerve—a long and complex cranial nerve, extending from the brain stem all the way down to the abdomen—is to keep the brakes of this stress response applied at most times and to release the brakes when we're facing a threat.

When the brakes come off, Wilson says, "Energy gets taken away from other neurological systems, including concentration, attention, rational problem-solving, immune response, metabolism—all those processes go offline." A high level of cortisol engages the parasympathetic nervous system (along with other neurochemical reactions), which helps our bodies to eventually reach a calmer state.

"That can't happen if the threat does not pass, if it's persistent," says Wilson. "If you're in a situation where you're experiencing ongoing harassment, you're having this constant activation of the sympathetic nervous system arousal ... and it can actually have a physical wear and tear on the body."

In her book *Girls on the Brink*, science journalist Donna Jackson Nakazawa explores the growing mental health crisis in adolescent females and provides an in-depth review of the evidence that girls' bodies respond differently to stressors than boys' bodies.

To recap what we learned from Chapter 3, as estrogen ramps up during puberty, its job is to promote the development of our body's organs and systems and to enhance the growth of neural connections in the brain—improving how different areas of the brain talk to each other and helping it run like a well-oiled machine. What Nakazawa discovered through her research is that the female brain at this time is more vulnerable and sensitive to outside threats because its job is to ensure the female's survival and that of her potential offspring. While research on sex hormones and stress response is still emerging, it would appear that social threats lead to an inflammatory response in the body, an "overpruning" of brain synapses (kind of like getting overenthusiastic with your hedge clippers), which drives higher rates of autoimmune disorders, anxiety, depression, and chronic pain in girls and women.

As Nakazawa contends, "This tells us that today's spike in chronic mental and physical health disorders among girls is a biologically rooted phenomenon: We have created a social-environmental landscape that may be altering the female stress-immune response in ways that turn on genes that derail thriving."[14] The key part of this to me is the "social-environmental landscape"—while Nakazawa sees the issue as being *rooted* in biology, she acknowledges that the *cause* is social. She's not arguing that girls' brains and bodies are inherently flawed; it is the unsafe and unequal world in which we raise girls that's causing these changes.

The social safety theory developed by George Slavich at the University of California, Los Angeles, gives some context here as well. Slavich hypothesizes that developing and maintaining friendly social bonds is a fundamental part of human behavior.[15] This means that threats to someone's social safety are the key stressors that affect our mental and physical health. For girls, Nakazawa argues that these threats are heightened in adolescence: "If you're getting, on the one hand, the constant message that, with one false step, you'll be cast out of the girl tribe and, on the other hand, that girls and women in general aren't safe in a sexist world, then you won't feel safe on any level. You're not entirely safe among your peers. And as a girl, you're certainly not safe on your own in our larger world. The stress-threat response never switches off."[16]

What's important to underline here is that Slavich contends that these responses to stress can, in many ways, be helpful. "It's all a way for our body, our minds, and our brains to adapt to circumstances we shouldn't be in," says Wilson.

The brains and bodies of girls and women have learned to adapt in the best ways they know how in order to cope with the ongoing threats they face. None of these ways of coping are "bad." Psychology might use the term "maladaptive," but I prefer to think of us doing the very best we can with the cards we've been dealt.

THE LINK BETWEEN SOCIAL CONFLICT AND EMOTIONAL SUFFERING

TO LEARN MORE about how mental illness is shaped by our social landscape, I connect with biocultural and evolutionary anthropologist Kristen Syme.

She points out that mental illness has a strong social component. "There's lots of cross-cultural evidence that psychological distress in general has an interpersonal aspect. As humans, we need our social group to survive more so than any other primate—more so than probably any other species," says Syme. Humans evolved in environments that posed significant threats, including starvation and disease, and working together meant the difference between life and death.

But "conflict and cooperation go hand in hand," says Syme. There are benefits in collectively defending ourselves against predators and sharing food and other resources, even if this close communal living can lead to frequent conflicts.[17] Neuroscience has theorized that this push-pull relationship is key to the regulation of our bodily resources, because our brain's primary job is to predict our biological needs before they even arise. Neuroscientist Lisa Feldman Barrett coined the term "body budget" to refer to the process by which our brain budgets our body's energy needs, monitoring things like cortisol, glucose, water, and salt. We feel good when our body budget is in balance, and we feel bad when it's out of balance. However, our brain is not operating alone: it's predicting our needs based on interactions with other brains around us.[18]

When our brain is in a loving and empathetic relationship with another brain, our bodies respond in a physical way, synchronizing heart rates and breathing patterns. In these cooperative situations, Feldman Barrett proposes that our brain will take fewer "withdrawals" from our body budget, and we get a chance to replenish our body's resources.

"A hateful word from a bully may cause your brain to predict a threat and flood your bloodstream with hormones, squandering precious resources from your body budget," writes Feldman Barrett.[19] Over time, harmful words or threats to our physical safety can lead to repeated withdrawals from our body budget, which result in a state of chronic stress. And as we've reviewed, girls and women are much more likely to face repeated threats to their emotional and physical safety.

It is this social conflict that Syme sees as a source of much emotional suffering, or what psychiatry would define as mental illness. Our suffering sometimes gives rise to behavior that our social group deems unbecoming. In the example of hysteria, women's socially undesirable behavior was almost always framed in relation to gender roles and sex—promiscuity, prostitution, and masturbation being three prime examples. To control these undesirable behaviors, women were coercively treated as mentally or physically ill by doctors who believed they knew best.

The evidence that Syme and her colleagues have gathered indicates that illnesses such as depression, PTSD, and anxiety are moderately heritable, are very common, and almost always manifest following adversity.[20] While specific neuro-developmental and mental disorders, such as autism and schizophrenia, are highly heritable and probably caused in large part by genetic variants, more common disorders could be better explained (and treated) by exploring an individual's history of adversity and social conflict.

"And it's not just adversity—it's adversity in the context of conflict," says Syme. Intense social conflict can include things like physical or sexual violence and harassment, marital or relationship conflict, and divorce. Syme's observations of many different societies around the world indicate that women bear the brunt of much of the social conflict we experience as humans. "It's not because women are flawed in some way that they have higher rates of depression; it's that women are more likely to be powerless, or to have less power relative to others around them," she says.

WHILE GROWING UP IN INDIA, Lasya Nadimpally didn't know anyone else who had divorced parents. With her father completely out of her life after she turned four, Lasya was raised by her mother's family. Divorce is a big taboo in Indian culture, and Lasya says she was emotionally and physically abused by her mother's extended family. "They didn't really understand how to handle this child out of divorce."

Lasya explains that her family was also extremely orthodox and closed-minded, which directly contrasted with the world outside her door in Hyderabad, a city of diverse religions and cultures. After she moved away from home to study journalism and communications, her friends became her primary family, filling in the relationship and support gaps that she had been missing since childhood. Despite a more stable life with school and friends, Lasya remembers specific triggers that would send her spiraling into depression and anxiety. She began talk therapy, something that is difficult to access in India and can cost a significant amount out of pocket.

While reading a book about mental health, Lasya filled out a quiz based on the adverse childhood experiences (ACE) study, which assesses different types of abuse, neglect, and trauma that children experience before the age of eighteen. "I scored six, and it was on a scale of ten," says Lasya. "When I was a lonely child who was getting beaten up every other day and I was just out of divorce and had lost half my family, nobody really cared to ask me how I was feeling."

A high ACE score has been linked to a significant number of health conditions, including heart disease and depression.[21] For any child, a higher ACE score is a major risk factor for future mental and physical health problems, but one study has shown that being female *and* having a high ACE score is riskier than either independent risk factor alone. In Nakazawa's book, the lead author of the study, Robert Whitaker, director of research at the Columbia-Bassett program at Columbia University, says, "One of the key possibilities is that because of discrimination, women and girls often experience their gender identity during development in ways that are traumatic."[22]

Lasya says that it took her many years to acknowledge the gender discrimination that she'd faced. "For the longest time, I thought I'd never grown up with any gender bias," she says. "Until one day... my grandmother told me, 'Your father left you because you were a girl.'" Lasya says she internalized that message, feeling an enormous pressure to succeed like a man would in the traditional patriarchal framework that equates success with money and status.

Lasya came to realize that many of the physical health issues she'd struggled with as a teen could be linked to her childhood experiences of abuse. She had a severe case of polycystic ovarian syndrome that wasn't detected until her mid-teen years and was instead treated as a problem of obesity. "The gynecologist used to be like, 'This is because you are fat,'" she says. Lasya was given diet pills and put on birth control at an early age. In college, she was diagnosed with type 2 diabetes and was advised that to avoid future health problems, she should consider bariatric surgery.

Lasya says that all these factors have had a major impact on her mental health. "There are so many voices in your head. And it becomes really difficult to recognize which one is yours and which one is objectively not yours."

For Lasya, healing has meant freeing herself from the myriad voices that have told her who she is. "I think my definition of healing has just become unlearning," she says. In the aftermath of her family violence, Lasya saw herself repeating patterns that drove her to misery, to the wrong kinds of people and the wrong life decisions. "I've never been able to prioritize my own self in my life," she says. "So I think healing has become more about how much in touch with my own self I am, and how authentic am I being to my own needs."

THE ANTIDOTE: HOW NOT TO GET RAPED, HARASSED, TOUCHED, OR HURT

LASYA'S STORY ILLUSTRATES how girls and women cope with violence and discrimination, the individual effects of which are social, physical, and psychological. There is evidence that trauma from sexual or physical violence disrupts neural activity in different parts of the brain's networks. Ruth Lanius, a professor of psychiatry and director of the PTSD research unit at Western University in Canada, has found that activity in the central autonomic network, which is responsible for regulating our heart rate, can become disconnected from actual heart rate measures in individuals who have experienced trauma. Normally, these systems work in unison, and the brain sends signals to the heart to influence heart rate variability. "Heart rate variability is really a marker of emotion regulation capacity, of how quickly you can adapt to different situations," Lanius says. "But the affected networks are also critical to cognitive functions such as focusing, memory, and planning, as well as a person's sense of self."[23]

These new neural pathways created after trauma or repeated stressors can make healing that much more difficult. Julie S. Lalonde is a survivor and women's rights activist who documents her harrowing story of intimate partner violence in the book *Resilience Is Futile: The Life and Death and Life of Julie S. Lalonde*.[24] "I think ongoing threats make it difficult for us as women and girls to even feel the changes in our body, because oftentimes it's the air we breathe," she says. "You don't question your behavior; you just sort of view it as a personality quirk—'I'm a very impatient person' or 'I'm not a good sleeper.'"

Without a single identifiable incident, women might not even be aware that they need to heal from anything. "The year after my stalker died, I was in the worst shape I've ever been mentally—I was constantly suicidal, I was very unwell, and I was confused by it," says Lalonde. Others in her life were confused as well, because the consensus was that the threat to Lalonde's safety—the man who had been stalking her for over a decade—was gone. She says that this emphasizes the *post*-traumatic part of it, in which a woman must process what's happened to her. "It feels impossible because these have been my coping skills and how I've moved through the world. It takes a long time to be able to parse out 'Who am I, apart from my trauma?'"

Lalonde says that in her work with thousands of survivors of sexual violence, she's seen many behaviors that help women cope. "We make ourselves smaller—literally and metaphorically, we try to take up less space," she says. Eating disorders are one of the well-documented results of abuse, but Lalonde has also observed that women are less likely to go out, to travel, or to take risks. These issues aren't acknowledged or talked about as much as behaviors like self-harm and substance abuse.

For some, stepping forward and seeking help comes with additional challenges beyond the gaslighting that many survivors face. In her book *What We Don't Talk About When We Talk About Fat*, Aubrey Gordon writes, "For all our talk about sexual assault being an act of power, not desire, as a fat woman I knew that those statements always came with caveats, asterisks, footnotes. I knew that my body was reliably withheld, an obvious exception to the rule. After all, we'd be grateful for whatever we got. *Who would want to rape us?*" Women who do not fit the standard Western mold of desirable and vulnerable (which is typically a white, thin, wealthier woman) are less likely to be believed or supported.[25]

Actor and longtime activist Jane Fonda, interviewed on the podcast *We Can Do Hard Things*, says that she thinks "sexual trauma and abuse causes women—it happens to men, too, but mostly women—to become disassociated from their bodies. It's very easy to slip away from a relationship to your body, especially for women because so much importance is put on our body." After being sexually abused as a child, Fonda says she went through much of her early life wanting to be perfect, because she believed that nobody was going to love her otherwise. Healing from that mindset, she says, was like seeing a double image in an eye exam come together. "I had to work really, really, really hard to bring myself back into myself," she says.[26]

Lalonde notes that women are often praised for their coping behaviors, reflecting a lack of understanding of what trauma can look like. "For me, I became a workaholic. And it became this really vicious cycle where it was also the place where I found purpose, and how I felt like I had worth in the world because I was doing things. And so if I stopped doing those things, then my self-esteem would plummet. I was just trying to stay busy so I didn't have to think about the dark thoughts in the back of my brain," she says.

Research would suggest that perfectionism, which is closely related to the behaviors Lalonde describes, has been increasing over time in Western countries and can be a trauma response. Whether these behaviors are associated with gender is still not clear. One meta-analysis by Thomas Curran and Andrew Hill included 41,641 American, Canadian, and British college students (around 70 percent female) in studies conducted between 1989 and 2016.[27] They found that levels of socially prescribed perfectionism—defined as doing things because you want others to perceive you as perfect—have linearly increased over time. Curran and

Hill describe this type of perfectionism as characterized by individuals believing their social context is very demanding, that others judge them harshly, and that they must display perfection to secure approval. For girls and women, I would argue that the site for this approval is often our bodies.

Socially prescribed perfectionism is the most debilitating of the three dimensions of perfectionism; the other two being self-oriented (setting impossibly high standards for yourself) and other-oriented (setting impossibly high expectations of others). When we assume others have impossibly high standards for us that we'll never meet, we can experience an increase in depressive symptoms and suicidal ideation. Curran and Hill write, "Broadly speaking, then, increasing levels of perfectionism might be considered symptomatic of the way in which young people are coping— to feel safe, connected, and of worth."[28]

Some studies show higher perfectionist tendencies for female adolescents or young adults, while others have not found a gender-based association.[29] What is apparent is that childhood experience of abuse (emotional, physical, or sexual) in girls predicts higher levels of socially prescribed perfectionism and a stronger drive to present a perfect image of herself to the outside world.[30] The motivation to be perfect might be either external or internal, but both forms can be maladaptive, meaning they lead to unhealthy thinking and behavior patterns (and ultimately mental distress).

Most of this research on perfectionism is in white Western populations, but a growing body of evidence can be found in different cultures and ethnicities. The research is mixed, but there is some evidence that socially prescribed perfectionism carries mental health risks across all cultural contexts, while other forms of perfectionism (e.g., the types often linked to pressures placed on kids by high-achieving parents or coaches) may show some differences.[31] It is difficult to assess cross-culturally because even within broad cultural categories (e.g., Asian-American), there are significant variations between families and individuals.

An influential paper by author Tema Okun argues that perfectionism is a function of white supremacy culture, in that the idea of being perfect is based in whiteness.[32] This characteristic of white supremacy culture values competition and individualism while seeing mistakes as a personal failing. While Okun's work is specific to schools, workplaces, and community-based organizations, others have made a similar link to wider cultural norms and ideas about women's value and worth in society.

As a white woman, I have recognized that perfectionism is rampant in my own culture; it feels like both an important strategy I've employed to face social threats *and* a driver for multiple (and often maladaptive) ways of coping, including diet culture, body shaming and fat bias, drug and alcohol use, and the grind culture of work. All these behaviors help many women to cope with the pressure to be "good" and to feel accepted—essentially, to feel safe. For me, addressing the mental health outcomes of perfectionism has meant facing the fact that patriarchy and white supremacy intersect—to be a "perfect" woman in our society is to be white, nondisabled, and attractive to men.

Some girls and women strive to meet Western society's ideal body type, and as in Jane Fonda's case, it can lead to disordered eating. If motherhood is in the cards, there can be a hyperfocus on "perfect" mothering to meet that expectation of the feminine ideal, which we'll discuss more in the next chapter. For those like Lasya and Lalonde, perfectionism shows up at work and striving to do more (and do better).

SMASHING THE PATRIARCHY IS NO EASY FEAT

IN THE STUDY on adverse childhood experiences by Robert Whitaker and colleagues, they conclude that treatments for depression and anxiety disorders in girls and women might be improved by addressing the joint impacts of developmental trauma and sexism. Although their study didn't include data on sexism, they say that their findings suggest that the stressors of sexism can be amplified by other childhood traumas in a way that makes the risk of these traumas *and* being female that much worse. "Therefore," they write, "treatments for depression and anxiety disorders in girls and women may be unsuccessful if they focus only or primarily on symptom management, with either medications or behavioral therapy."[33] Treatments need to address what it means to be a girl or woman in our society and explore how rigid gender norms and discrimination worsen mental health outcomes.

Granted, these kinds of solutions are focused on the individual, and that's what many programs or treatments target—changing girls' or women's behaviors to help protect them from harm or to treat stress and trauma after it's happened. I ask Helen Wilson what she sees as solutions to sex- and gender-based violence. "Just based on my own observations, I think interventions tend to be very superficial and driven from legalistic requirements," she says.

For example, encouraging women to report sexual assault, submit to a forensic medical exam, and release this evidence to police can have legal consequences for perpetrators (granted, most prosecutions do not result in sentencing, which is a whole other issue). Ultimately, though, targeting women's behaviors doesn't change the underlying reasons that women are being sexually assaulted in the first place. Treating chronic stress and trauma should include *preventing* sexual violence from happening.

Lalonde says she doesn't disagree with this, but that interventions that target women are still valuable. "I don't just mean physical defense," she says. She reminds me that most violence is perpetrated by someone close to a woman, which means it's not always about "stranger danger." Women need to understand the warning signs that partners are becoming abusive, such as a partner isolating a woman from her wider social circle and community. "I push back against this feminist narrative that teaching self-defense or teaching women about red flags is regressive and victim blaming and puts the onus on women," says Lalonde.

Both Lalonde and Wilson tell me about a rape resistance program developed by Charlene Senn at the University of Windsor, the only program available that's been evaluated in a clinical trial. Participants learn about healthy relationships, physical and verbal self-defense strategies, and empowerment techniques. Women who participated in the twelve-hour training had a significantly reduced risk of rape or sexual assault over the two-year follow-up period.[34]

As a trained child psychologist, Wilson also feels that early development is critical—teaching children in early life about how to show consent and respect for others. This, she says, goes beyond basic sexual education to normalize consensual, respectful relationships.

Teaching consent or addressing misogyny with boys and men sounds like an important strategy, but Lalonde tells me that not a single program to date has been proven to work. "What we need is a tremendous amount of research into finding something that does work with men," she says. And research requires funding, which is already in short supply when it comes to women's health.

INSTEAD OF DIAGNOSING WOMEN as mentally ill, I would love to see a world in which we diagnose our own society as disordered and turn our attention to the structures of power that have serious consequences for women's emotional health. "Smashing the patriarchy" means giving voice to women's stories and redefining a more accessible feminist agenda that recognizes that all women are not experiencing sex- and gender-based violence in the same ways. There is clear value in targeting women specifically with treatments or programs that reduce threats to their safety and help them to cope with trauma, but a multipronged approach is needed. Women, especially those who experience marginalization, require greater access to economic resources, and we need to better understand the ways that gender and cultural norms strengthen or weaken women's power.

But before we get too far into that radical work, we need to address the other elephant in the room, which colludes with patriarchy and, in some ways, is more difficult to uncover and identify.

7

ARE YOU MENTALLY ILL OR MENTALLY OVERLOADED?

Capitalism uses patriarchy as a lever to attain its
objectives, while at the same time reinforcing it.
DENISE COMANNE[1]

GROWING UP IN an upper-middle-class white family, I was
raised to believe that I could have it all—if I just worked
hard enough. I could get the best grades, be accepted into
any university, complete a master's degree, and find a high-
paying job in a field of my choice, while *also* having babies
and raising a family. I believed this narrative even when a
mental breakdown stopped me in my tracks and worsening
mental health continued to cloud my path through young
adulthood. I pushed forward because I felt that failure was
not an option. In my early thirties, I devoured Sheryl Sand-
berg's *Lean In* and became convinced that the multitude of
responsibilities I was carrying wasn't the source of my stress.

I had just not found the right technique to game the system. Life felt like a marathon that I was running with a toddler on each hip, while others passed me on the track with far less weight. I felt immense frustration that I was trying my hardest and couldn't run any faster.

An invisible backpack holds all the social pressures we carry as girls, women, and, especially, mothers. In her book *Fed Up: Emotional Labor, Women, and the Way Forward*, author Gemma Hartley describes the historical trajectory of the concept of emotional labor (or what some of us call "mental load") and expands its definition to "emotion management and life management combined. It is the unpaid, invisible work we do to keep those around us comfortable and happy."[2] In other words, it is the cognitive and physical work that occurs within a household *and* a workplace, as well as the mentally exhausting job of managing the emotional lives of others—the burdens of caregiving and the emotional intelligence we are expected to develop to meet the needs of others. Another term that's used is the "worry work" that women do, anticipating the needs of those around them and acting to manage those needs throughout the day and week.

Mental load has been studied within sociological and feminist fields of research, with much of the literature centering on cognitive and physical labor in relation to household management. This is made up of the everyday mundane tasks that keep our homes and families functional: managing homework and activity schedules, taking an aging parent to medical appointments or providing care for them, washing and folding clothes, feeding the children (who are bottomless snack pits), caring for pets, and putting away the Lego pieces that threaten the delicate sole of your foot. It is in this work that the gender revolution has stalled out, with studies showing that even during pandemic lockdowns where both partners were home, women were responsible for more unpaid housework than their male partners.[3]

Researchers in social and political sciences at the University of Melbourne qualify three components that make up the mental load:

1. It is invisible and therefore difficult to quantify.

2. It is boundaryless; mental load spills over into every aspect of our lives in the workplace, at home, and in leisure time.

3. It never ends; there is no "clocking out" from mental load.[4]

Almost everyone engages in cognitive labor, which is how we think, plan, and troubleshoot issues of household management, and it can be balanced with the needs of our working roles. In research, cognitive labor is measured through surveys and time-use studies, which have people self-report and track every hour of their time throughout a typical day. The shortfall in these methods is that they don't account for the invisible mental load. Surveys ask questions about how much time we spend on housework and paid work, which suggests there's a clear line we cross when we leave the home and head to work. This doesn't address the mental burden that women carry in every setting; there's no "off switch" to hit as soon as we're traveling to work. To begin tackling the social and structural issues of mental load, the first step is to make it visible by measuring it.[5]

I tried a self-help version of this one day to illustrate for my husband exactly what happened throughout my day. (I later read the book *Fair Play* by Eve Rodsky, and she suggested a similar activity—and yes, I recognize the irony in using self-help for a problem that's not of my own making.)[6] My desire to document these tasks followed an argument in which I'd (once again) brought up the fact that I felt overwhelmed by the mental load I was carrying. To give credit where credit is due, my husband listened and really tried to understand the gist of the problem. But his response—"Just ask me to do something and I will!"—was not what I was looking for.

I began by listing off all the worries that popped into my head the minute my eyes opened in the morning—the dreaded to-do list and tasks that I had forgotten from the previous day. Then it was the physical and emotional work of getting two children out of bed and off to school, breakfast and lunches made, the dog walked, until I collapsed in my chair at the office at 9:30 a.m., feeling as though I had already lived an entire day.

The mental load continued from there. Instead of logging "work time," I was continually interrupted throughout my day with tasks that I had to complete. Here's a sampling of that list:

- Birthday party this Saturday; send RSVP; need gift for birthday party.

- Realize bills are due. Pay hydro and gas bills online.

- Receive email from school: outing next week, they forgot to send out the email so could we please approve online ASAP. Oh, and they need volunteers.

- Check schedule to see if I have time to volunteer for outing.

- Text message from Mom: "I want to give your dad his birthday present this weekend; can we arrange a shared Skype call?" Back and forth for ten minutes on the best time to Skype.

- Respond to emails about a friend's party. Organize food.

- Sign up for parent/teacher interviews.

- Add school outing and interview dates on to family calendar.

- Try to work.

- Read email from child's theater teacher.

- RSVP for child's birthday party.

- Work.

- More texts from Mom about day/time for a call.

- Add Dad's call to Google calendar.

- Remember to add credit card bill due dates into Reminders app.

There are two entries for work time in this list, and although I didn't track how long they lasted, I'm sure that they weren't overly productive. This pattern meant that I was usually trying to catch up on work in the evenings.

In the end, I didn't even finish the list and never shared it with my husband. It felt petty somehow, and I realized that an open conversation when we were both calm and receptive was a better bet. We have had many such conversations over the years, and this ongoing communication helped to change our relationship and flag for each other when life was becoming overwhelming for either of us. And to be clear, my husband carried the load as a stay-at-home parent for a period and genuinely understood the pressures I was facing managing the household. The problem was that when both of us worked full-time, the bulk of the emotional labor often fell to me.

What I was inexpertly and unscientifically trying to create with my list was a robust and standardized measure of mental load. No such measure yet exists, but if one did, researchers could use it to track the problem in different countries and among different populations. We need to know how much time women spend on mental load (hint: all day and night), where they are tackling the mental load, and how it's shared between partners or other family members. This information could then be used to develop effective interventions at the individual and the family-unit levels, and it could inform broader policy changes.

The connections between mental load, stress, burnout, and mental illness are all still a bit murky, but I think this is an important piece of the puzzle of why so many girls and women struggle with mental illness. Stick with me while I review some of the literature on mental load and burnout, and then I'll propose how I think they're linked to mental illness.

"IF MEN WERE WILLING to step up more, to acknowledge the many roles women are expected to play, and to voluntarily, willingly, and genuinely carry some of that load, we would have a very different dynamic," says Taslim Alani-Verjee, a psychologist, founder of the Silm Centre for Mental Health in Toronto, and cofounder of Feelings Unpacked. "There is a possibility for that dynamic to change—but it doesn't, because those who have the power aren't willing to give it up."

Scholars Jean Duncombe and Dennis Marsden argue that achieving gender equality (in what I assume to be hetero-sexual relationships) for the cognitive part of mental load is likely feasible.[7] Since the publication of their work in the mid-1990s, there is evidence that men are doing more of their share of household tasks, although a fairly wide gap remains. In the U.S., women spend around four hours a day on unpaid work compared to 2.5 hours for men.[8] Chores still tend to divide down gender lines, with men doing more out-door work and car repair and women doing more cooking, cleaning, and indoor work. (Obviously this is generalized across the population—I know many women who change their own tires and do tons of yard work.)

The bigger and much more difficult task to achieve, say Duncombe and Marsden, is to equally divide the emotional work, or what they call "the problem with no name."[9] They conclude that any changes made to achieve greater equal-ity with respect to mental load must address heterosexual men's "masculine identity," which has traditionally been emotion-phobic and strongly tied to economic goals, like earning an income.

As I proposed in earlier chapters, women are not inher-ently more emotional and thus better suited to emotional labor; it's that our culture *believes* we are, and we perpetu-ate this myth through the ways that we socialize children to take on different responsibilities in the home and in the public sphere. In white Western culture, particularly, girls and women are taught that the way to deal with mental load and gender inequality is to lean in harder and work faster. Not only is this problematic, but I would argue it is also making us mentally unwell.

Racialized women and women from marginalized ethnicities carry a complicated mental load, which often extends beyond the individual or family unit. "We represent the entirety of our race or ethnicity or culture," says Alani-Verjee, "and so then not only do we carry the load of our family unit or community—if one person is suffering, we're all suffering. Every battle feels personal, and every battle feels like if we just sit back and let it happen, that we're letting people down.

"We can never, ever ignore the social and systemic factors that affect mental health," she continues. "Because it's inaccurate and it erases the hardship, the struggle, the courage, the resilience—it erases all of it to not think about mental load in a systemic way." However, Alani-Verjee adds that the *consequences* are certainly individual, and the ways that we each internalize the problem look very different. "I think part of it is to acknowledge that mental load and stress can vary and are almost always heavier or higher for racialized and marginalized people."

For LGBTQ+ individuals, some data suggests that the mental load may be shared more equally in relationships. Research has shown that lesbian couples divide household tasks more equally than heterosexual couples and also have better communication in tackling this divide.[10] However, when LGBTQ+ couples have children, they divide tasks just as heterosexual couples do.

This would suggest that our roles are about more than a gender divide; our society and workplaces have been built around a capitalist ideal: a full-time worker and a stay-at-home partner. As Abbie Goldberg, a psychology professor at Clark University, explains in a *New York Times* article, the idea that same-sex relationships are an "egalitarian utopia" where emotional labor is divided equally is overly simplified.[11] If kids come along, there's still an invisible part of cognitive labor that's unaccounted for.

Mental load is messy to track and to address—it's not a straightforward household-management or relationship problem. It's also economic, in how our society values different kinds of work and how the modern workplace operates. And when the workload becomes too much, women are more likely to be the ones who burn out.

CONNECTING THE DOTS: MENTAL LOAD, BURNOUT, AND THE IDEAL WOMAN

"TODAY'S WORKPLACE THINKS and operates much as it did in the 1950s, when people expected the world to be neatly divided into two separate and unequal worlds: the man in the gray flannel suit who could devote himself entirely to work in one, and, in the other, his homemaker wife, taking care of everything and everyone else," writes Brigid Schulte, author of *Overwhelmed: Work, Love, and Play When No One Has the Time*.[12] However, this idyllic portrait of work-home life was always a myth, reserved mostly for upper-middle-class white families but never the reality for lower-middle-class and working-class families and women from racialized communities.

"For most women, the luxury of being a housewife, simply caring for children, cooking and cleaning and creating a peaceful haven for the hard-worked husband who brought home the bread at the end of the day, was only ever an illusion created by the middle classes," writes researcher Amanda Wilkinson for *The Guardian*. Wilkinson's research has revealed that most women in the nineteenth and early twentieth centuries held nontraditional working roles in agriculture, warehouses, and manufacturing.[13]

The heady days of the 1950s in suburban North America seem to be a bit of a blip in our historical understanding of women and work. The 1950s and subsequent feminist revolution also painted a picture of choice, which has spilled over into our twenty-first-century conversations about "working moms" versus "stay-at-home moms," as though somehow everyone can freely choose which camp to join if they start a family. Dig a little deeper, and you'll find that some of the "choices" we make about work are a result of social pressures women face and the rigidity and inflexibility of the modern workplace. Often, it feels less like a choice and more like we're just getting pushed out.

This transitional postwar time also created a popular professional persona, what Schulte calls the "ideal worker"— the individual who puts in eighty-hour workweeks and eats, sleeps, and breathes work (likely they're not doing much actual sleeping and eating).[14] Western capitalist culture continues to idolize this kind of dedication, and we champion it as if it's a model for success, especially for men and fathers. In the modern economy, the "ideal worker" and "ideal woman" have blended together, with specific gendered expectations for work and home life.

"When we imagine the 'ideal feminine woman,' she is a caregiver, she is strong, assertive, but also loving and warm, and is the person people can come to. She is emotionally available all the time, and can juggle it all, in a way that men are never ever expected to do," says Alani-Verjee. "Even when we can recognize the impossibility of being that woman, it's still the version that comes to our mind of success ... we still try so hard to be a version of that, to fit with our values and beliefs and identity." Because the ideal woman is the benchmark, it always seems like we're failing, says Alani-Verjee.

"If you're a nurse, a teacher, or a mother, particularly, we love to pay lip service to these people, but we don't give a shit what we pay them," says Bethany Johnson, coauthor of the book *You're Doing It Wrong! Mothering, Media, and Medical Expertise.* "You're supposed to feel good about your job because it's a nice thing to do." She points out that once middle-class women were encouraged to work full-time after second-wave feminism, they weren't offered resources or help for dealing with the mental load. "A lot of people are also struggling because our expectations have gone up for what mothering looks like and what having a family looks like and what the family unit is responsible for doing," she says.

So, wealthier families invest in private tutoring, schedule swimming and music lessons, purchase ecofriendly products and organic food, and insist their children learn two languages, all in the name of providing them with a super-enriched childhood experience that mothers are usually tasked with managing and organizing. This has been dubbed "intensive mothering," which some researchers suggest could be something that perpetuates traditional gender roles.[15] And while none of those activities are inherently "bad," intensive mothering on the whole benefits men by absolving them from doing a lot of the unpaid emotional work. There are also socioeconomic implications, as the bulk of this intensive mothering is carried out by wealthier women in heterosexual relationships; women with less financial power may feel similar pressures but face greater barriers to achieving the idyllic family life that wealthier women present on social media and blogs.[16]

What's more, increased pressure to maintain intensive mothering leaves many women exhausted and on the brink of burnout. It's a form of burnout that arises just as much in the home as it does in the workplace.

TAMMY B. (not the same Tammy that you met in Chapter 4) is an elementary school teacher in the U.K. Prior to the pandemic, Tammy was working in a school with students who were primarily from underserved communities. "Across the board, the culture was to work through the evenings and through the weekends, which is very typical for most teachers around the world," says Tammy. "And that's fine, I think, when you are on your own, or it's just you and another partner, but then my wife and I had twins, and at that point life got really, really busy."

When one of her twin girls was diagnosed with hearing difficulties and required several operations, Tammy felt that her work performance began to slip. She would miss a meeting or email and found it difficult to keep things running smoothly. "At that point, I started to lose my confidence in how well I could perform in the role," she says. On the heels of this came her elderly mother's illness, and Tammy was frequently traveling five hours north to care for her mother before her death. "I had a couple of talks with supportive colleagues, and I remember them saying that it feels like you can't be a mom at work, and you can't be a teacher at home, so you end up being neither. But the reality is that you're all the things."

While Tammy was grieving the death of her mother, her employer gave her one month's paid leave and then adjusted her workload when she returned, scaling back her responsibilities to allow her more time with her family. But even with those adaptations, Tammy felt like her passion had gone from the job. "It's not something you can fake with children, and it just felt like things weren't going well," she says. "But I didn't know I had a problem—I was probably the last to see it."

It was the head teacher at the school who suggested Tammy should take a longer break and start mental health counseling, and when Tammy returned home that evening and announced her departure from her job, her wife was not shocked. She had witnessed the worsening emotional exhaustion and pointed out that Tammy had not been acting like her usual self. Normally quite a patient person, Tammy found she lost her temper with the kids, often over small things. "That wasn't the parent I wanted to be," she says.

In much of the medical literature, burnout has been studied as it relates to our adult working roles; a clear line in the sand is drawn between who we are as employees, managers, or entrepreneurs and who we are in the home. The latest revision of the International Classification of Diseases (ICD-11) states that burnout is a phenomenon with three defining characteristics: emotional exhaustion, a sense of detachment from one's role (or what is called "depersonalization"), and reduced productivity in the workplace. This means that, at least within our medical understanding, we aren't meant to apply the concept of burnout to our lives outside an occupational context.[17]

I would argue that this makes the concept of burnout—both our cultural understanding and treatment of it—a largely capitalist one. The notion that individuals can "heal" from burnout in order to jump right back into their jobs fails to address the root cause of the problem. There is a fundamental truth that burnout for women is about more than discovering "work-life balance" or tackling inequality in the workplace—it's also about the mental load (both cognitive and emotional) and how it spills over into our working lives.

In a large cross-sectional study of 2,026 workers from Canada, a deeper exploration of the gendered pathways that lead to burnout identified that women had lower levels of decision latitude, which means they have socially limited access to control and power within the workplace. Women also experienced higher work-to-family conflict, which could mean they struggled more with their recovery from burnout. Strategies to reduce burnout included women investing more time outside the workplace (perhaps through part-time work arrangements), in work from home, and in nonwork activities like childcare and household responsibilities.[18]

The authors cautioned that while these strategies may help women to feel better, reducing time spent on work activities can lead to fewer career opportunities and likely exacerbates gender inequality in the workplace. This observation isn't intended to put more pressure on women to set higher goals or to work harder. Instead, it highlights the reality of the modern workplace: less "face time" at the office often means fewer opportunities to get noticed, fewer promotions, and weaker relationships with managers and coworkers.[19]

Tammy says her time in therapy helped her to realize that her job was not sustainable for her in the long term. She didn't know if she wanted to change careers, but she had to face the fact that the way she had been giving all of herself to her role had led, in some part, to her burnout. "My therapist called me a people pleaser," says Tammy. "Possibly what helps me teach is that I always want to help the students; I always want to fix things. And for an employer, not being able to say no to things is actually a gift to them, because then I'll take on more tasks."

Tammy's comment about being a "people pleaser" gave me pause. It's something I personally identify with, and I hear the same label time and again from many women in my life. Returning to the concept of social safety from Chapter 6, I strongly suspect that many girls grow up motivated to respond to social safety threats by being "good"—if we are good, then it's less likely we will be cast out or hurt in some way. And to be "good" is to please others by always saying yes.

In a piece on people-pleasing for the *Washington Post*, Allyson Chiu sums up the thoughts of interviewee Natalie Lue, author of the book *The Joy of Saying No*: "Women, in particular, have long been expected to suppress their own needs and cater to others ... while people in minority groups may face pressures to work hard, perform and be 'the model minority.'"[20]

A set of experiments conducted with undergraduate students at the University of Pittsburgh illustrated how women are expected to cater to others. A computer randomly created mixed-gender groups of three people who were tasked with getting one group member to volunteer to click a button, without using any form of communication. (Each student was seated at their own computer, and all decisions were anonymous.) If no one volunteered to click the button, everyone in the group received $1. If someone volunteered, the volunteer received $1.25 while the other two group members each received $2. This continued for ten decision rounds.

Lo and behold, women were 48 percent more likely to volunteer compared to the men. The researchers hypothesized that women volunteered more because others expected them to. To test this, they reran the experiment with the groups made up of only men or only women. In this case, the all-men and all-women groups ended up having the same success rates in finding a volunteer to click the button and take the pay cut. The researchers concluded that it isn't that women *like* to take on extra tasks (often menial jobs that no one else wants to do!); it's that there's a social expectation that women will always step up.[21]

TAMMY'S EXPERIENCE ILLUSTRATES the overlapping relationship between burnout and mental illness, which researchers are still trying to tease out. There does seem to be a strong link between burnout, depression, and anxiety, but no conclusive evidence that one causes another.[22] One study of nurses found that participants with significant levels of burnout were more likely to screen positive for any mental disorder, particularly major depressive disorder.[23]

In a study of Finnish employees that measured biomarkers of physiological stress (called "allostatic load") and depression, the authors found that burnout was indeed putting strain on the body, but that depression explained 60 percent of this association—which means there was a lot of overlap. The study suggests that the association between burnout and depression is likely two-way: burned-out people may be more likely to become depressed, and depressed people are more vulnerable to burnout. However, the path from burnout to depression appears to be stronger.[24]

When women are experiencing burnout in a more general "I'm so exhausted with everything" sense, it is sometimes diagnosed as anxiety or depression. The authors of a 2019 review caution that the similarities between burnout and depression or anxiety could lead to a false diagnosis and that burnout itself might be overlooked.[25] When this happens, treatment solutions may prove ineffective, leading to worsening symptoms or an abandonment of treatment altogether. Treatment for mental illness generally centers on therapy and medication; treatment for burnout would likely encompass more holistic solutions, like time off work to rest, negotiating different working hours with an employer, and self-care strategies including sleep hygiene and exercise. Of course, treatments for these conditions overlap in many ways, but treating burnout as mental illness may mean that the underlying economic and social issues women face are not being addressed.

Though it's speculative, I would like readers to consider something: What if the high rates of anxiety and depression among women are, in large part, caused by burnout? What if the reason you can't get out of bed is more about the world you live in, the job you hold (or no longer hold), and the power you lack rather than about *you* as a person? Personally, this realization completely changed the way I relate to myself and my mental illness. I believe that misdiagnosing burnout feeds the illusion that mental illness is due to a personality flaw, negative mindset, my family's genes, or an imbalance in my brain rather than an understanding that is closer to the truth: I'm facing a social problem that has real, lived emotional consequences. For some, this realization may be distressing: it means acknowledging that you don't have as much control over your well-being as you once thought. But I hope that some of you find this freeing, that it lifts the veil shrouding mental illness and sets you on a path to rediscover your own capacity, the ways in which you are limited, and what tiny acts of resistance you can make.

FED UP: THE PUSH AGAINST MENTAL LOAD AND THE RISE OF SELF-CARE

IN MY OWN LIFE, I knew that something had to change, but I was at a complete loss as to what that might look like. I'd tried the time-management apps, I had a giant calendar posted on the wall, I tried to get enough sleep at night and squeezed in a workout when I could find the time. I also had the money to invest in "self-care" like massage, yoga classes, and healthy food. But it seemed like the harder I worked to manage it all, the less successful I was; it never occurred to me that the system was rigged to ensure my defeat. What I have come to realize is that the whitewashed and consumerist version of self-care many of us are sold is directly tied to an idea of individual, self-determined happiness and mental and physical wellness—which ignores the biopsychosocial factors that make us unwell in the first place.

Although "self-care" has become a buzzword in the past decade, its roots can be found in the early twentieth century, as a medical or public health concept that encouraged patients to take better care of their physical health.[26] Guidelines and public health campaigns target self-care components of lifestyle (e.g., smoking, alcohol consumption, eating habits, and exercise) with the aim to help people reduce disease or mortality. But the problem is that (save for smoking) it's been difficult to prove that changing one or two discrete behaviors can impact the overall health of an individual.[27] Furthermore, this approach ignores the social and economic factors that have a much greater influence on our health and well-being. One widely cited study estimates that social determinants of health, including things like poverty, employment, and education, account for 47 percent of health outcomes, whereas individual health behaviors make up 34 percent and clinical care influences 16 percent.[28]

Take obesity, for example: there is no good evidence that being overweight or obese (as defined by the highly flawed body mass index or BMI) is an *independent* predictor of poor health outcomes, like higher mortality.[29] Yet every year billions of dollars are poured into research and public health campaigns, which tell people to manage their weight through "self-care" activities like diet—though no diet has ever been proven to be effective for weight loss over the long term.[30]

Self-care hasn't always been so narrowly defined. When the women's and civil rights movements took hold in the 1960s and 1970s, self-care was conceived of as a radical political act, a way for marginalized groups to reclaim their bodies and disrupt white supremacy and patriarchy. Juxtaposed with these movements, wellness trends in wealthier communities began to weasel their way into mainstream culture. This flavor of self-care was less about surviving and more about thriving—if you had the money to actually improve your quality of life.[31]

Because of stigma, early public health lifestyle campaigns never tackled mental health. These days, the focus of these campaigns is largely on individual self-care behaviors that are thought to improve overall physical *and* mental health. Employee wellness programs and public health departments instruct us to practice deep breathing, exercise, and find "balance" in our work and home lives. The self-care messaging for women in particular has changed in the past century, from the earlier promotion of relationship-oriented activities (maintaining our home and families) to activities that encourage us to become strong, self-made individuals. By focusing on ourselves as worthy of love, we can supposedly achieve more and be happier and healthier.[32]

It sounds like a lovely sentiment, but it's often couched in consumerist self-care rules, from "wellness" rituals like eating whole foods and creating workout calendars to purchasing specific clothing or products. Gwyneth Paltrow's entire Goop empire revolves around the belief that women can walk a healthier and more successful path in life by working on the self (both the body and mind) rather than engaging in social action that would change power structures and systems.[33] While Goop is one of the more extreme examples, subtler messaging can be observed in many online spaces that cater to women. And often, these messages replace important medical advice or treatment.

Wealthier (and often white) individuals encourage women to manage their energy stores by pursuing what *You're Doing It Wrong!* coauthors Bethany Johnson and Margaret M. Quinlan call more "feminine endeavors": "to have a positive, sunny outlook, and to remain cognizant of stress, anxiety, and nervous strain"—advice that's rampant in feminized health challenges like infertility.[34] This type of practice is a by-product of the era of hysteria, when it was believed that emotional or nervous distress caused systemic dysfunction in the body. It's certainly easier to sell the self-care message than it is to provide adequate medical care for health issues.

"There's this big gap between the type of health care you can get if you're a super-resourced person, and the type that you get when you aren't, and this drives a lot of people to social media because they're trying to fill in this gap," says Johnson. Wellness influencers on social media have capitalized on this need for proper health care, and it feeds into the phenomenon I discussed in the introduction: White Woman Wellness Syndrome.

"It's all about the double binds we get put in," says Quinlan. "We end up getting stressed out doing all the things we're told we're supposed to do to reduce stress, because we are unable to change the structural issues that would give us more time, money, and resources to be able to 'de-stress.'"

Johnson and Quinlan say that women are repeatedly targeted with the message to "reduce stress," which reinforces the idea of our gender as hyper-emotional; we can then blame the problem on the individual rather than on the minimal research and support that is available for women's health, mothering, and care work.

"What happens to people's mental health when they're told all of their stress and all of the structural issues they battle are all in their head?" says Johnson. "Why would you *not* become clinically depressed as a result of that?"

Our culture's modern understanding of self-care has gendered implications, with most of the focus on individualized behaviors that we task women with (on top of the unequal and unpaid labor they are already responsible for)—all in the name of achieving a "perfect" state of mental and physical health. This commercialized brand of self-care is largely futile and can exacerbate anxiety and depression.

THERE'S A WAY TO IMAGINE self-care as an authentic and meaningful practice that contributes to better health for individuals *and* communities. Taslim Alani-Verjee says that it's helpful to think about authentic self-care as comprising several different parts: there's the basic self-care that we need to do daily, like brushing our teeth, moving our bodies, and eating (yes, just eating, rather than constantly striving toward some type of eating). Then there are the pampering activities, like a massage, bubble bath, or eating out at a nice restaurant, which is where the modern self-care industry has thrived. Finally, self-care can sometimes be about caring for other people within our community. "I think the self-care culture is really individual," she says. "What feels good for many of us is taking care of others, and that's not bad or wrong self-care."

Alani-Verjee also says that there's a whole layer of the conversation about self-care that's often missing, which is that we all have many different facets—spiritual, social or relational, cognitive, emotional, and financial. "When we can split it up that way, we realize there are so many things that we may or may not be doing to take care of ourselves. It's about recognizing that we're more than just bubble baths and baking; we have to invest in all parts of ourselves."

This means there is no "should" in self-care—it's highly individual, and it may take some practice to figure out what works best. For you, self-care might mean attending a religious service or spending time in nature. For someone else, it's catching up on bills or finally creating a budget to deal with debt. Social self-care might be spending time with a good friend who provides you with comfort and laughter. Emotional self-care could be therapy if that's accessible to you, journaling, or resting quietly for ten minutes during the workday. The self-care industry wants you to believe that it's about buying more things to make yourself "healthier," but it's actually very basic activities (and often non-activities) that lead to greater strength and capacity to withstand the exhausting systems we live in.

"I NOW UNDERSTAND that my mental health is a constant; it's not a poor thing, it's not a great thing, but it's checking in with yourself," says Tammy. "How are you feeling today, and what's something you can do in your day that will help?"

Following the advice of her employer, Tammy took twelve weeks' paid leave and received eight weeks of counseling through the U.K.'s National Health Service. Week by week, Tammy and her counselor deconstructed her burnout, focusing on the parts of her life that were nonnegotiable (like family) and the parts where adjustments could be made. Her therapist suggested that she visit her family doctor, who recommended sleeping pills in the hopes that they could avoid prescribing an antidepressant. Tammy's sleep patterns were disrupted by high levels of stress, and she struggled to fall asleep and stay asleep through the night. The pills helped in the short term, and Tammy worked with her counselor to implement healthier sleep habits, like limiting caffeine to the mornings, observing regular sleep times, and turning off technology to wind down before bed.

She eventually returned to her previous role full-time, but after the pandemic hit, she knew she needed another change. The role Tammy ultimately landed was in a special-needs school for boys, which concentrates on mental health and recovery.

"With the boys, we do a lot of work in nature and the forest, and do more practical activities," she says. "I don't have thirty books to mark in every lesson, every night, and when I'm finished at six o'clock, I go home."

Not giving all of ourselves to fill the rest of the world's demands is about boundaries—how we stop the relentless flow of energy that leaks from our bodies, as though we're sieves and not solid human beings. As Tammy and I wrap up our conversation about her burnout, she shares a story about a recent meeting of her school's leadership team. Tammy was the only woman in the room, and one of her male colleagues turned to her and asked her to take the meeting minutes. She replied, "No, actually, I'm going to pass on that, thank you," with no explanation or justification. She doesn't think that four years ago, before her burnout, she would have been able to set that boundary.

Boundaries are scary to implement, and I don't know about you, but I never *feel* good when I'm enacting them. I'm always thankful in the weeks and months after I've forged a boundary, but the "in the moment" act of telling someone no, of being honest about my limits, provokes an icky feeling. Our gendered socialization teaches us to give without limits, to expect nothing in return, and to bury ourselves in the process.

Saying no is the primary way that I've begun my own private revolt against mental load. It's obviously not the only solution, but I've come to realize that unlike personal health and wellness, workplace culture, and gender norms, saying no is fully under my control.

THE SOLUTIONS

WE NEED TO EXPAND our definition of burnout beyond the workplace and start to take stock of the invisible mental load that may be contributing to women's overall state of exhaustion. We can't separate work and home life because it is all "work." And what's more, the emotional work that occurs in all life contexts is undervalued, is unpaid, and may be contributing disproportionately to the higher rates of mental illness that we are observing among women. Understanding emotional labor as tethered to mental health can change how we define the problem and how we try to fix it.

At its core, burnout is a mismatch between our body's resources and the world's demands, which makes it a social issue with emotional consequences. To prescribe a medical or consumer-oriented self-care model as the treatment allows us to ignore the structural problems that set us up to fail. "To make it individual is to take the politics out of it," says Alani-Verjee. "I think society benefits from women being in this role."

Yael Schonbrun is a psychologist and assistant professor at Brown University, and she sees that burnout is related to an unavoidable conflict between roles and demands, in that we all desire to be engaged in work that we love to do and simultaneously be deeply engaged in family life.[35] From an evolutionary perspective, Schonbrun says that our brains are wired to care for others in larger groups rather than small family units. In higher-resourced countries like the U.S. and Canada, our culture has veered off in a completely different direction—deciding the family unit should be able to do it all, with the man as the practical/financial head and the woman as the emotional head. "It's a very weird society we live in," says Schonbrun. When individuals inevitably reach the point in their parenting journeys where they realize they can't manage everything on their own, Schonbrun says that guilt becomes an additional burden. People who aren't parents but provide care for family members or friends may also reach this point, especially in cultures where there is little outside caregiving support.

"Concepts like alloparenting can help us to unhook from the guilt and say... what I'm experiencing is so normal," says Schonbrun. "Alloparenting" is the anthropological term for the communal care of children, which has historically been evenly distributed to many different people in a child's life—grandparents, aunties, uncles, cousins, and neighbors.[36] I would extend this concept to caregiving in general, so that providing support to a close family member (say, an aging parent) doesn't fall on a single individual but is a communal responsibility. With the help of paid providers, close friends, and other family members, caregiving burdens can be lessened.

A big problem for many families, like mine, is that we are geographically removed from our extended family members, having left our "village" for better job opportunities. Modern alloparents now fill the void, but these are often paid providers, such as daycare and social workers, teachers, and therapists. What the COVID-19 pandemic revealed is that these alloparents are not, as Schonbrun and Rebecca

Schrag Hershberg write in an article for *Behavioral Scientist*, "a nice-to-have, [but] a have-to-have."[37]

Which means we need to find ways for all parents (and nonparents as well, especially those who care for other family members) to have access to communal care, whether we're able to pay for it or not. Universal childcare and better-quality elder care are a good start when it comes to public policy, because leaving the burden on women to patch together a network of alloparents is ineffective. This "free system" completely broke down during the pandemic, and mental load researchers argue that we need to learn from this situation in the post-pandemic world.[38] As the population ages and many of us find ourselves sandwiched between caring for children and aging parents, the problem of mental load will only place additional strain on women.

At the same time, women could grow old waiting for these policy shifts (and in some countries they are likely to wait much longer), so there is something to be said for patching together extra supports. Schonbrun argues that women can get creative in their local communities, forging connections with neighbors and accessing free resources through local community centers. This strategy links back to the idea of self-care as community care—that all of us deserve support in shouldering the burdens of caring work.

Devon Price, a social psychologist, professor, and the author of *Laziness Does Not Exist*, says expanded worker protections make it easier for individuals to say no to exploitation and guilt, and to attain better work-life balance. "We need better assurances for workers with disabilities, and guaranteed leave for parents who have just had kids, because here in the United States such things are not guaranteed and the people who suffer the most from the lack of such services are the most marginalized among us," he says.

Saying no and setting boundaries, in Price's opinion, need to be done collectively. "Otherwise, many of us will risk getting fired, demoted, kicked out of our housing, kicked out of educational programs, and more. I really think joint efforts such as unionizing, collective bargaining, and more organized, intentional 'quiet quitting' is important, in addition to all the personal self-advocacy that can help individuals in the short term," he says.

The more I've learned about burnout and mental load, the more I've started to make small acts of resistance to push back against capitalism and, by extension, patriarchy. Some of my thinking around this topic has been inspired by Tricia Hersey, the founder of the Nap Ministry and author of the book *Rest Is Resistance: A Manifesto.*[39] Hersey's organization and her book reintroduce the radical aspect of self-care and urge us to take up rest as a form of resistance, because it disrupts and pushes back against capitalism and white supremacy, which go hand in hand. There is a well-documented link between the slave trade and the development of capitalism in North America.[40]

Hersey writes, "Many people believe grind culture is this pie-in-the-sky monster directing our every move, when in reality, we become grind culture. We are grind culture."[41] In order for capitalism and white supremacy to continue to thrive, we all need to keep feeding the system, through the false belief that productivity is the answer. Hersey encourages her readers and followers to take up the gauntlet by resting and napping. It sounds silly on the surface, but reading deeper, the act of rest can liberate people from oppressive systems.

While reading Hersey's book, I recalled a recent experience I had at a spa. A coworker had given me a generous gift card, which I put off using for almost a year. I finally booked a facial, which was an hour-and-a-half ritual of cooling creams, facial massage, and hot towels. I slept the entire time, drifting in and out of consciousness as the esthetician did her thing. After I left, I had a good laugh with my husband that I had just paid someone $150 so I could take a nap. Why is it so hard for me to walk away from my desk at home and lie down in my own bed?

It is, I think, the dominant social and gender norms that make it seem like I need *permission* to rest, and yet there's no one to ask for permission. Like Hersey says, there's no "monster" in the sky or man behind the curtain. We all live in and through this system, and that's why it continues to function the way it does.

I'm not suggesting that every individual can fix racism, oppression, and gender inequality simply by taking a nap (and if you read Hersey's book, you'll understand the deeper message behind rest). However, I do think that through collective acts of resistance—stepping back to let others volunteer, making time for rest, or saying no—we can begin to restore our sense of agency in our own lives. We can also be like Toto in *The Wizard of Oz* and pull back the curtain to see the truth of the systems in which we live.

I'm still a work in progress when it comes to rest. Even though I now recognize the way that patriarchy, capitalism, and white supremacy keep me and many other women stuck in a cycle of burnout, I continue to struggle with disrupting these systems because they are so *compelling* (no surprise there, since I, too, benefit from these systems). I could come up with dozens of excuses at this moment as to why I can't take a break from writing and close my eyes for twenty minutes.

What has helped me push the needle forward on this is to consider rest as not the opposite of work. In a popular TEDx Talk, Saundra Dalton-Smith identifies seven domains of rest: mental, spiritual, emotional, social, sensory, creative, and physical. She asks us to consider which domains we're drawing energy from throughout our day through different tasks—for example, commuting to work might take energy from our mental and sensory buckets.

Our rest deficit is where we're using up most of our energy throughout our day. Dalton-Smith says our job is to focus our attention on which types of rest we truly need to restore each of those seven areas. If getting more rest for you means sleeping more (which is often the advice health care providers give to burned-out people), or maybe scrolling on your phone for two hours, then Dalton-Smith argues that you will be chronically tired, because neither of these activities are filling up all your buckets of rest.[42]

Physical rest is about naps, but it might also be about changing your workspace, so that you're not standing or sitting too long. Mental rest is when you get to "zone out" (and this could be combined with creative rest, because many creative activities lead to a flow state when you're attending to a task, like doodling, painting, or any other activity that you fancy).[43] For me, sensory and social rest are about having quiet time to myself, turning off fluorescent lighting, and minimizing online meetings, which I find draining. By incorporating rest throughout my entire day, I've come to see this practice as integral to my personal sense of agency.

It also leaves me with energy to fight for better, and to extend support to women facing greater burdens than I am.

WE HAVE SEEN THAT burnout and mental load are strongly linked to mental distress and are placing great strain on women's capacity to function in systems of power, where there are widely differing levels of privilege and disadvantage. Burnout is both an emotional and a social problem and results from accumulated stress in any sphere of our life, whether this involves paid or unpaid work. Furthermore, burnout may be misdiagnosed as mental illness, which could mean that the treatments being offered are exacerbating the problem. Wider system change is well overdue, but in the everyday time crunch of our lives, individually focused solutions can help provide women with some small relief from carrying a too-heavy load.

In the next two chapters, I'll investigate the most common treatments offered to women experiencing mental distress, and why these may not always be the fix we hope for.

8

THE PROMISES (AND PITFALLS) OF THERAPY

Much will be gained if we succeed in transforming your hysterical misery into common unhappiness.
JOSEF BREUER AND SIGMUND FREUD¹

FOR PEOPLE SUFFERING from more common types of mental illness, talk therapy (often along with medication) is considered a first-line treatment. Many Western countries have publicly funded talk therapy services, even though it's usually the more severe cases that get bumped to the front of the line. Others wait weeks, or sometimes months, to get in the door.

After going through my teenage breakdown, I was referred to a child psychologist at a local hospital, and I finally felt some relief knowing that help was at my fingertips. The anticipation of someone else taking control immediately boosted my mood, and because it was the late 1990s, wait times for mental health services were reasonable. I was in the door within a month.

My psychologist worked out of the local hospital psychiatry unit in a shoebox of a room with a worn couch and desk. Light struggled through one small foggy window, which faced the sidewalk above us.

"It's nice to meet you, Misty," he said. "You can call me Jeff." His voice was gentle but confident, and I immediately felt at ease. I had been imagining a stern bespectacled man with a white beard, who would look intensely into my eyes and ask me to tell him about my relationship with my mother. Given the era in which I grew up, the ideas I had about therapy had been shaped by television and movies, with a Freudian chaise longue and dream analysis. I was about to discover a new world of talk therapy, one that focused entirely on the present and my everyday challenges.

In many conversations I've had with women about their treatment and recovery, there is always one person who stands out—that one doctor, nurse, or counselor who listened well, who helped facilitate new insights and cocreated new paths to better living and healing. We carry these people in our hearts, and we hear their voices in times of stress. Jeff was that person for me, and he pulled me out of my burning house just in time. Over the year we spent together in that cramped office, Jeff never pushed me where I didn't want to go, and he patiently helped me work through my mental health crisis.

Jeff and I spent our time together exploring the iceberg of fears I had floating below the surface. In particular, cognitive behavioral therapy (CBT) worked well for my high-strung personality, encouraging me to challenge unrealistic beliefs and pull myself from spiraling panic. First, I would lay out my fears in a long list, and together we would examine the thoughts behind my worries.

Situation: Boarding a packed train with friends for a night out on the town.

Thought #1: I will be trapped. (Emotions: fear, panic)

Thought #2: People will see I'm having a panic attack. (Emotions: shame, embarrassment)

In the next step, Jeff would ask me to challenge those thoughts. He'd pull out his trusty notepad and jot down my thoughts, then pass the notebook to me to write down my counterthoughts:

Counterthought #1: I'm not trapped, because I can get off the train at any stop.

Counterthought #2: My friends care about me. If they see me struggling, they will be there to help.

We also discussed different types of thoughts, such as black-and-white thinking, overgeneralization, catastrophizing, and labeling. The thoughts that dominated my mind could be packaged up into neat little thinking styles—most of which were fueling my anxiety, Jeff proposed—and these needed to be challenged for me to develop a healthier thought process. My thinking pattern was also fueling extreme perfectionism as I fought to maintain high grades, participate in multiple extracurriculars, be a reliable employee, and maintain a busy social life. For many years, I had pushed myself to the limits of what I could achieve and felt unrelenting pressure to meet (what I imagined were) the very high expectations of me.

TALK HAPPY: CBT AND
OTHER TALK THERAPIES

WHILE BIOLOGICAL PSYCHIATRY and psychoanalysis dominated the field of mental health treatment in the mid-twentieth century, cognitive psychologists and behaviorists attempted to have their voices heard as a valid alternative. Once staunch rivals, the cognitive and behavioral agitators came together to form the most popular and well-studied treatment for depression and other mood disorders: cognitive behavioral therapy.[2] Widespread adoption of these techniques, and years of research, have proven that the approach holds significant value in the treatment of mental illness. In a large overview in 2012 of 269 meta-analyses examining the efficacy of CBT, the authors concluded that "the evidence-base of CBT is very strong."[3] However, they did caution that more randomized controlled trials were needed and that evidence was lacking for racialized groups and people of low socioeconomic status.

The premise for most talk therapy is simple: the patient and therapist talk, thought patterns and behaviors are explored (and sometimes challenged), and the patient comes out of the process with better "thinking tools" for coping with adversity.

"CBT is more of a foundational approach to therapy, where the therapist is the expert, and you teach the client strategies, skills, and coping mechanisms," says Lindsey Boes, a marriage and family therapist whom you met back in Chapter 5. "It's very formulated, and there's a reason that there are so many studies over the decades showing that CBT works—because it's manualized." This provides consistency, and scientific study of a therapy that can be applied in the same way in any setting generally gives more solid and dependable evidence.

CBT doesn't ignore physical feelings, but the therapist helps to break down problems into separate parts: the anxious thought ("I'm scared that I'll faint"), the physical sensations ("My heart pounds and my hands get sweaty"), and the action ("I leave the situation as quickly as possible"). The goal is to change the thought, which creates a domino effect of changing the physical sensations and behaviors. CBT is very much focused on the here and now, so there's no exploration of past relationships, trauma, or family dynamics (with the exception of CBT therapies that have been adapted to focus on trauma). It also doesn't address wider societal or environmental problems that may be affecting a person's well-being.

People all around the globe and many of the women I spoke to for this book have received CBT or other forms of talk therapy and found it helpful. However, there may be some limitations. In a meta-analysis of CBT for treating substance use, the authors found only a few studies that were able to engage and retain Black and Hispanic participants, which is consistent with existing research looking at the effectiveness of CBT for non-white participants.[4] Dropouts in trials happen for a variety of reasons, but this study suggests that there could be a conflict between the needs of some Black or Hispanic populations and the way that CBT plays out in practice. The researchers also state that "the limited inclusion of women in clinical trials is alarming" and could indicate specific barriers that prevent racialized women from accessing CBT for substance use (which was the focus of their analysis). Possible explanations include a lack of transportation or childcare, distrust of the medical system, fear and shame, the belief they can recover without help, and a general lack of knowledge about the services that are available.[5]

There is also evidence that CBT might not lead to longer-term improvement in some mental disorders. A meta-analysis from 2021 looked at the efficacy of CBT and another talk therapy, called psychodynamic-interpersonal therapy (PIT), for individuals with eating disorders (the majority of whom are female). They found that CBT was the most effective, with about one-third of the included patients, and one-half of those with bulimia, in remission after going through therapy. But based on their analysis, the authors suggest that the therapy itself (changing eating disordered thoughts and behaviors) might not have led to remission. It appeared that other factors, including personal motivation, better cognitive ability, and lower rates of pre-existing depression, played a greater role in remission than the talk therapy itself.[6]

Research on the efficacy of CBT for those who are neurodivergent is also lacking. One study that examined CBT for younger individuals diagnosed with autism spectrum disorders (ASD) and co-occurring obsessive-compulsive disorders (OCD) showed promising results, though individuals with ASD often require modifications for CBT, including the use of visuals, positive reinforcement, and clear language and instructions.[7] In the adult population, a few randomized controlled trials have been conducted looking at CBT alone or with medication to treat people diagnosed with ADHD, and these have shown positive results.[8]

One of the moderators here is the length of treatment—most trials are analyzing short-term efficacy of CBT (over eight to twelve weeks of therapy). One review found positive outcomes over the long term, but a substantial number of participants in their sample did not improve following treatment and a smaller number experienced worsening symptoms.[9]

For Lindsey Boes, CBT is helpful when she has a client who's having a hard time understanding their actions. They want a very tangible answer for their behavior—to identify the thought that triggered a reaction. But with many clients, Boes prefers narrative therapy, an approach that aims to reduce the restraints of unhelpful stories about ourselves created by dominant power structures. "Narrative therapy is very postmodern, in terms of believing the client is the expert in their own life, not the therapist," she says. "There are steps to make CBT more culturally sound, but addressing someone's sociocultural environment is not inherent in the philosophy behind the therapy itself." Boes gives me an example of a queer Black woman who comes to her for therapy because she's experiencing a lot of anxiety and fear in public. If Boes uses CBT to teach her to challenge those feelings, she's overlooking the fact that the woman often isn't safe in the world and that fear and anxiety function to help keep her safe.

"We need to separate the problem from you," she says. "I've had clients talk about anxiety or depression as chaos, the dark cloud, or—my favorite—the porcupine." It then becomes easier to set boundaries with something that isn't tied up with a person's identity.

Women especially need to detach their self from mental illness, because the narrative for so long has been that our minds and bodies are the problem.

AFTER DOING A FULL YEAR OF CBT with Jeff, I felt cautious and hopeful that I could leave my problems back in high school, along with bad boyfriends and questionable life choices. During my last appointment, Jeff congratulated me on all my hard work and then said in his gentle voice: "Many people who deal with these issues as teens go on to deal with them again in adulthood. It's something you should prepare for." I nodded in agreement but secretly didn't believe him. I had mastered my thoughts! Overcome my panic! I almost wanted a therapy certificate with a shiny *A* for "amazing."

But I soon discovered that Jeff was right. Despite my significant achievements in tackling the thought processes behind my panic attacks, stable mental health was not something that would come easily to me. I was initially optimistic after leaving Jeff's care (and leaving child psychology to enter mainstream adult services), but my anxiety and depression symptoms did indeed rear their ugly heads at various times throughout early adulthood; and when they did, CBT became less and less effective for me.

Katherine, whom you met in Chapter 4, also cycled in and out of different types of talk therapy after experiencing her first mental health issues at the age of twelve. She saw several care providers throughout her twenties, and she's been seeing her current therapist for over three years. "I feel like because I've had ongoing issues, long-term therapy is what I need," she says. Developing a deeper relationship with a therapist has helped Katherine's depressive episodes shorten and become less severe.

She remembers trying CBT once with a psychiatrist, but for her, the process felt very distant from the heart of the problem. Intriguingly, Katherine saw her mental health issues as more internal and felt that CBT was addressing something external. "I felt like CBT was more about changing your thinking... but the depression is coming from inside me—it's not about the things going on outside," she says. She concedes now that she recognizes external stressors in her life, but at the time, she located the *feelings* of depression deep inside her body. "CBT just didn't feel like the right approach."

Katherine is not the first woman to tell me that CBT wasn't as effective for her as everyone makes it out to be. In my own experience, CBT was a great starting point when I was in a crisis situation. It was later, when I began to desire an approach that would address all the pressures I faced as a woman living in Western society, that I found talk therapy fell short.

HEALING WITHIN THE BODY

THEORIES HAVE SURFACED in the last few decades that the way humans heal from adversity is not typically by thinking our way out but primarily within and through our bodies.[10] This relates to growing scientific understanding of the mind-body connection (or, if you recall the discussion in Chapter 5, what many understand to be a brain-body connection).

Neurological research has proven that there are networks in the cerebral cortex (the largest area of your brain) that connect to the adrenal medulla, the inner part of the adrenal gland located above each kidney. The adrenal medullas are responsible for the body's stress response—our pounding heart, sweaty palms, and dilated pupils—which prepares our body to fight or hightail it out of a stressful situation.[11]

In *ScienceDaily*, the author of a published study, Peter Strick, says that this connection "raises the possibility that activity in these cortical areas when you re-imagine an error, or beat yourself up over a mistake, or think about a traumatic event, results in descending signals that influence the adrenal medulla in just the same way as the actual event."[12]

This could also help to explain why body movement, like yoga or tai chi, is so helpful in moderating the stress response, because the connection between the cortex and adrenal medulla centers in a region of the spinal cord that controls our "core" muscles and the regulation of the sympathetic nervous system.

"We can all create more room, and more opportunities for growth, in our nervous system. But we do this primarily through what our *bodies* experience and do—not through what we think or realize or cognitively figure out," writes Resmaa Menakem in his groundbreaking book on racialized trauma.[13]

People who have experienced trauma or other repeated stressors may at times feel almost entirely disconnected from their bodily experience, but they can also report severe physical symptoms.[14] Research shows that among survivors of interpersonal violence, women report physical symptoms more frequently than men.[15] These symptoms might include chronic pain, gastrointestinal issues, or heart problems. While some might say that trauma is "stored" or "trapped" within the body, I suspect that a more scientifically correct phrasing would be that trauma "manifests" in the body, sometimes as a numbed-out feeling and other times as intense physical sensations. As I've argued in this book, girls and women are at a much greater risk of experiencing trauma and a dysregulated stress response, which makes it imperative that we better understand the mind-body connection and the interventions that could interrupt a stress response.

While I don't necessarily place myself in the category of a person with trauma, I do see that the ways I had been experiencing and coping with stress since early childhood had elements of a traumatic response. Looking back, I realize that there have been very few times in my life when I was not afraid; I was incessantly on high alert, my body likely flooded with cortisol, my heart hammering.

Trauma is not always related to a single catastrophic event, like a car crash or natural disaster; it can accrue over time and be caused by a series of smaller events that disrupt the ways in which our bodies respond to stress. This is called complex PTSD, which the DSM-5 does not recognize, but the International Classification of Diseases 11 (ICD-11) names the condition and its impact on emotional regulation, self-identity, and relationship with others.[16]

Most treatments for PTSD and trauma rely primarily on CBT and exposure-based methods. Exposure therapy aims to help an individual overcome their fears by confronting the thing that makes them scared—but this is done in small increments with the support of a safe person.[17] However, people who suffer from trauma show impaired cognitive functioning, which means they are sometimes unable to think their way through their trauma responses. As well, exposure can often be terrifying and confrontational, and it can exacerbate symptoms rather than making them better.[18]

Body-based practices such as massage, occupational therapy, or yoga—which we can do on our own or with trained practitioners—target the body directly. As we covered earlier in this chapter, narrative-based approaches like talk therapy use language to better understand our thoughts and mental landscape. A relatively new approach gaining traction within therapeutic communities combines both of these strategies in a framework called somatic reappraisal, which deals with both levels of emotion processing—the body and the mind—to help a person heal from mental distress.[19] This framework offers an alternative technique for women who have not responded well to traditional CBT methods.

The first part of the practice involves bringing our attention to our inner body experience—the beat of our heart, the tightness in our muscles, our stomach gurgling, and the rise and fall of our breath—which is known as interoception.[20] By building up our awareness of these sensations, we can learn to better understand the granularity of emotion, which allows us to expand beyond the narrow definition of "good" or "bad" that we often use to describe our feelings.

One promising treatment on the horizon that could aid in the process of interoception is called flotation-REST. For this treatment, you enter a tank of water saturated with Epsom salts, which allows you to float unaided. There is no light or sound in the tank, which reduces demand on the nervous system and makes you more aware of your breathing and heartbeat. Preliminary data from one trial found that a one-hour tank session had short-term anti-anxiety and antidepressant effects, likely related to the reduction of sensory input, which appears to help us focus more closely on the body's sensations.[21]

Once we've learned to observe our bodily sensations and attend to them, the second part of somatic reappraisal has us become aware of the story we tell ourselves about what these sensations mean. This is the narrative part of the process. The stories our brain tells and the language we use about our bodies can shape the way we're feeling. A flutter in the stomach might be labeled as "excitement" by one person and "anxiety" by another. Maladaptive narratives about sensory information happen when we interpret a sensation as negative, and then we repeat this process over and over until we are stuck in a negative pattern of feeling and thinking. Somatic reappraisal helps us learn to tell ourselves a new story.

Cynthia Price, a research professor in the School of Nursing at the University of Washington, developed a specialized treatment approach based on this theory, called mindful awareness in body-oriented therapy (MABT), which is designed to teach people somatic reappraisal skills that can be used at home and in everyday life.[22] In an email exchange, Price wrote to me that her research on women with substance use disorders has shown that they have continued to practice body-based strategies (which make use of somatic reappraisal) long after the therapeutic intervention ended.

Somatic Experiencing is a similar therapeutic approach developed to meet the needs of people for whom CBT has a limited effect; it's also considered as a complement to the CBT- and exposure-based methods already proven to work for many individuals. This trademarked therapy uses a technique called "bottom-up processing," which guides an individual's attention toward our internal, bodily landscape, including our sensations, movements, and actions within the body and within the space around us.[23] One review of Somatic Experiencing found promising results, but the overall quality of the included studies was mixed.

As is usually the case when evaluating alternative treatment options, there is a need for more trials that are properly conducted to meet quality standards.[24]

There is evidence that the process of looking inward and practicing mindful awareness of the body creates measurable changes in the brain.[25] To learn about these changes, I spoke with Cortland Dahl, a research scientist with the Center for Healthy Minds at the University of Wisconsin–Madison and an expert on mindfulness. "The main principle of neuroplasticity is that the brain is constantly changing based on experience," he says. "Over time, those brain networks can be strengthened or weakened depending on what you do." By focusing our attention on breathing or other internal bodily sensations, over time we can induce changes in the brain that may propel us toward more adaptive coping strategies, as well as a better understanding of ourselves and of the sociocultural forces working on and around us. Somatic reappraisal isn't just fanciful thinking—it's changing our brains *and* our minds, which eventually changes how we experience and manage emotions.

REFRAMING OUR EMOTIONS

FIRST, A QUICK RECAP on emotions research from Chapter 2, because I think it's important to understand this in relation to body-based therapies: the consensus among cognitive and psychological researchers up until about a decade ago was that emotions depend on a trigger, or "stimulus."[26] Something happens in the world (for example, you see someone crying), which triggers a specific emotion (sadness) in one area of your brain. This earlier research is based on the belief that there are commonalities in emotional expression that all humans recognize. Anger is shown in a grimace, sadness as a frown, and happiness is a smile. But new research has called into question the idea of universal emotions.

What some neuroscientists now propose is that emotions are constructed through our brain's complex network of neurons, and they happen because our brain is trying to keep us alive, not because something has triggered us to feel them.[27]

I'll tell you a little story of how this works and why I think it is so important to the therapeutic techniques we provide for girls and women who are struggling with mental health challenges. Recently, one of our neighbors experienced a fire that produced loud explosions, thick smoke, and lots of ash. Since that day, anytime my daughter sees smoke or fumes (even if they're not related to a fire) or hears a siren wail, she becomes terrified.

When my daughter's brain attempts to make meaning of what she's hearing or seeing, it's using information from the body to predict what the body needs to protect itself from danger. These predictions occur all day and night without our conscious awareness, and sometimes, like in the case of my daughter's conception of fire, the predictions are wrong.

"Every thought, memory, perception, or emotion that you construct includes something about the state of your body: a little piece of interoception," writes neuroscientist Lisa Feldman Barrett.[28] Our brain must do something with these sensations and makes meanings from them. If my daughter spots a puff of white gas floating by, the brain regions that manage her body have *already started* to increase her heart rate and divert blood flow to the muscles. Her brain then registers those physical sensations and predicts that she is seeing fire and should prepare to run. These predictions turn into emotions of fear or terror.[29]

When I hug my daughter and soothe her by saying, "Don't worry, it's just some fog," her body budget needs to recalibrate. Because this system is a bit slow on the uptake, it takes time for my daughter to calm down. Our prediction system gets things wrong over and over again, and our bodies can become depleted—essentially, we are in the red and we end up feeling mentally and physically worn down.[30] Though it's speculative, I would argue that this is what is happening to girls and women who have faced real threats in the past; the brain is making predictions of *future* threats, which may not always be correct.

Our brains are perceiving moment-by-moment signals from the body, and it's at this point that the cognitive mind kicks in—it's not the simple thought-feeling-action sequence that CBT proposes. The awareness of all these internal sensory signals allows women to subjectively figure out what their bodies are trying to tell them, and—no surprise to those of you who have experienced panic attacks or anxiety— the mind can be a poor judge of sensory character.[31] People with anxiety, depression, and panic often have poor body literacy skills, which means they find it hard to accurately interpret sensory signals.

Physical sensations in the body and our understanding of what they mean are shaped in large part by our culture. Kristen Lindquist, whom you met back in Chapter 2, uses the example of hunger, the physical sensation that I personally experience as low energy, shaking hands, agitation, and eventually, if I don't get any food in me, feeling "hangry"—with an overwhelming anger that causes me to lash out at my unsuspecting family. (My husband is now so used to this behavior that he notices the signs first, brings me a snack, and commands me to eat.) "Evidence is mounting that women have a unique experience of hunger, caused by how we filter our own biology through gendered concepts about the body," write Lindquist and colleague Mallory Feldman in an article for *Aeon*. They reference mounting evidence that women can be poor evaluators of changes in our physiology, which means that we either ignore bodily sensations (a numbed-out feeling, which is more common in women who have experienced trauma) or we mistake a sensation for something else (like how I think I'm really angry when I'm just hungry).[32]

This mistake is also the result of self-objectification, which is when women view their bodies as objects separate from themselves. Internalized misogyny means we understand that our bodies are primarily valued for their outward appearance. "There is a huge focus on girls' bodies, but it's completely external, and not internal," says Lindquist. "There's so little focus on their own experiences and their own appraisals of the world." The more we experience self-objectification, the less capable we are of detecting our own internal physiological cues. This is likely linked to the higher incidence of dieting and eating disorders among girls and women and in the LGBTQ+ community.[33]

Neuroimaging studies of the brain have found that a region known as the insula is responsible for creating meaning about our body's condition. The rear and middle insula receive messages of physical sensation from the nervous system and spinal cord; these messages are then projected forward to the front of the insula, where we become conscious of the sensation—like a handy weather gauge that tells us if it's cold, warm, stormy, or gloriously sunny. Insula activation is associated with greater interoceptive sensitivity, which is how skilled we are at recognizing and understanding our physiological cues.[34] When our culture applies its own meaning and strict rules to our bodies, it becomes much harder for us to successfully detect these inner bodily changes and apply an appropriate meaning to the sensations that we do notice.

This is why it's so important for girls and women to become detectives of their own bodily experience and get more curious about how their brain applies meaning to feelings or sensations. As Cynthia Price and her colleague Helen Weng write in a paper on somatic reappraisal, "qualitative studies indicate the importance of interoceptive awareness practice for increased self-agency, embodiment, and skills for processing and coping with challenging emotions."[35]

Healing from anxiety, depression, and trauma largely depends on how we reframe emotional experiences, but in a way that taps into the body-mind connection rather than simply replacing "bad" thoughts with more helpful ones. In this way, girls and women can learn to reappraise their thoughts and bodily sensations together, usually through a bottom-up process of recognizing physical sensations together with thoughts that arise about those sensations.

THERAPY, WHETHER IT USES traditional talk or body-based approaches, is enormously helpful. However, our examination of structural and social issues has shown us that many women can't afford or access the therapy they need, and if they do happen to receive publicly funded therapy, it's often short term and doesn't address the social factors of mental health. When therapy is not an option or there are long waitlists, many doctors recommend medication. And it might come as no surprise by this point in the book, but there is strong evidence for gender bias in the prescription of mental health medications.

9

THERE'S A
PILL FOR THAT

Jesus loves me, this I know.
For he gave me Lexapro.
GLENNON DOYLE¹

"THINK OF IT LIKE THIS," my doctor said. "You wouldn't feel
bad about taking insulin if you had diabetes, right? This is
the same situation, but you need medication to help your
brain function in a better way."

Sitting in the plastic chair in the examination room at
my doctor's office, I listened to this familiar refrain with a
sense of defeat. I rolled a tissue in my hands over and over
until tiny bits of it sprinkled down on my legs like snow. I
had managed to keep my composure until I began explaining all my symptoms to the doctor, and then the floodgates
had opened.

I knew I was in a bad place. The year of therapy with Jeff
had built the essential groundwork for tackling some of the
learned habits I had developed in relation to my anxiety and

depression. CBT had helped me make progress, but it wasn't enough to prevent relapses that led to months of rebuilding my confidence and my drive to heal and recover.

At twenty-five years old, I had finally flown the coop and landed in Toronto to complete my master's degree. Seven years had passed since I first walked into Jeff's office, but some days I still felt as though I was at square one when it came to my mental health. Panic attacks were a thing of the past, but I'd funneled my anxiety into body image issues and disordered eating, perhaps the inevitable consequence of years of fear related to eating and the gastrointestinal symptoms that always followed. By this time, I'd received a second official diagnosis: "eating disorder not otherwise specified" (now referred to as "other specified feeding or eating disorders" in the DSM-5). I didn't fit into the neat symptom criteria for anorexia or bulimia. I chose compulsive exercise and extreme dieting, followed closely by binge eating, shame, and weight gain.

I was done fighting with what felt like extreme behavior and moods and had opened myself up to the offer of medication. The first drug I tried was called Effexor, a serotonin-norepinephrine reuptake inhibitor (SNRI) that increases levels of both serotonin and norepinephrine, neurotransmitters thought to support mood. These small pills packed a powerful punch in my anxiety-riddled brain, allowing me to sleep soundly for the first time in many years. I soon had an infinite capacity for sleep, dozing off during car rides and taking two-hour naps in the afternoon. My doctor suggested I take the medication at night to deal with the sleepiness, but I wasn't bothered by the side effect. In fact, I rejoiced in my new slumber habit after a decade of intermittent insomnia. The intense highs and lows in mood I had experienced now settled somewhere in a mellow middle, and I was able to move through the world with a level of indifference. I still cared about things, but it was as if someone had handed me binoculars and I could watch myself from a calm distance. Rather than getting caught up in the spiral of worry and panic, I felt my fears fall away like pieces of armor that I had been encased in for so long. What was left were feelings of confidence and capability, freedom, and ease.

But I soon discovered that wouldn't last.

THE PILLS THAT WERE
SUPPOSED TO END MENTAL ILLNESS

ANTIDEPRESSANTS, WHICH INCLUDE SNRIS, selective serotonin reuptake inhibitors (SSRIs), tricyclic antidepressants (TCAs), and monoamine oxidase inhibitors (MAOIs), are drugs that act on our brain's neurotransmitters. A neurotransmitter is a chemical that allows the nervous system to transmit messages between neurons or from neurons to other cells in our bodies (for example, our muscles).[2] These little messengers (which I like to think of as happy fellas with newsie caps, high britches, and a can-do attitude) are found not only in the brain but all over the body, including in the gut (more on this in Chapter 11). They are involved in many bodily functions, including digestion, sleep, and mood. SSRIs and SNRIS are the more commonly prescribed antidepressants, and they work on the brain by stopping the removal of specific neurotransmitters from the synapse (the structure that permits neurons to pass signals to other neurons) after they're released. That is thought to increase overall levels of the chemical in the synapse.

Around the world, consumption of psychotropic medication in the past twenty years has risen for all age groups, with the most significant increase being among women. Psychotropics are used to treat mental illnesses (and sometimes physical illness) and include antidepressants, anti-anxiety medications (Ativan, for example), stimulants (such as Ritalin), antipsychotics, and mood stabilizers. Between 2000 and 2015, the consumption of antidepressant drugs doubled in OECD countries.[3] The highest consumption per capita was found in Iceland, Australia, Portugal, the United Kingdom, Sweden, Canada, and Belgium.[4] In the U.S. between 2015 and 2018, 13 percent of people over the age of eighteen reported taking antidepressant medication, with women twice as likely to be consuming antidepressants compared with men. For American women over sixty, the rate of antidepressant use is even higher, at 24 percent.[5] On the other side of the globe, one in six Australians (over 18 percent of the population) filled a mental-health-related prescription in 2020–2021, with a higher proportion of them female than male (around 22 percent versus 15 percent).[6]

While some argue that the reason for this increased use of antidepressants is that the stigma and shame of mental illness and its treatment has eased, there is no clear data to support this theory. Stigma surrounding medication use for mental illness is still a big barrier to treatment, and many people report being unwilling or ashamed to take medication. Access to treatment is another hurdle to overcome, with white women far surpassing other ethnic and racialized female groups in the consumption of antidepressants. Data collected from 2015 to 2018 in the U.S. shows that 22.3 percent of white women had used antidepressant medication in the previous thirty days compared to 10 percent of Black women, 8.9 percent of Latina women, and 3.4 percent of Asian women.[7] This could relate to the stigma of mental illness and treatment within certain cultures but could also signal a bias in prescription practices.

Another proposed explanation for the rising usage rates of these medications is that there's a growing proportion of patients receiving long-term antidepressant treatment.[8] It appears that more of us are taking antidepressants for longer periods of time, with most prescriptions signed by family doctors and not by psychiatrists or nonpsychiatrist specialists.[9] With heavy caseloads and a lack of specialist training, general practitioners may lack the time to follow up or provide effective support for managing antidepressant use. Not everyone needs to stay on medication forever, but it appears that a lot of us are being left to manage our own treatment over the long term.

There has also been a growing movement to study the effects of antidepressants and whether these pills have actually delivered what they first promised—that they would be miracle drugs that relieve depression and other mental illnesses. "We do know that antidepressants are more effective than a placebo," says Simone Vigod, chief of psychiatry at Women's College Hospital in Toronto. "About two-thirds of people respond to the first medication prescribed." But among those patients who don't, the proportion who respond to a second or third medication drops. Eventually clinicians may need to explore alternative options, some of which involve adding other mental health medications. "No treatment has 100 percent effectiveness," Vigod says, which is "a thing that we as humans don't like very much—it's not very settling."

Around 60 percent of people respond to antidepressant treatment within two months, with about a 50 percent reduction in symptoms. However, one systematic review that analyzed twenty-one different antidepressants found higher dropout rates due to side effects compared to a placebo—patients taking antidepressants were consistently at greater odds of leaving the study due to adverse events.[10] The lead author of this review told *The Guardian* that "about 80% of people stop antidepressants within a month," but it's difficult to know if this is because patients were bothered by side effects or because they weren't seeing an improvement in symptoms.[11] Antidepressants take time to start working, and if patients in a trial suspected they had been given a placebo instead of the active drug, they may have decided to quit.[12] Based on this (and other) data, the Royal College of Psychiatrists in the U.K. have clarified that antidepressants work well for moderate to severe depression but not as well for milder symptoms.[13]

"I THINK ONE of the biggest things that finding a good set of meds did for me was to firmly plant a feeling of what 'good' can feel like," writes Kendra Pendolino, a woman from the U.S. who connected with me over Twitter after I asked for women to share their positive experiences with antidepressants. "I've had the deep depressions where my brain says that happiness is a myth that can never happen, that joy is unobtainable, that suffering is all there is," she continues, "and *after* meds, I experienced good, stable, fulfilling times." Though those times were not flawless or painless, they were sprinkled with laughter, happiness, and satisfaction. "Now that I've experienced that, it's a lot easier to tell my brain, 'Things suck right now, but they won't forever,'" she writes. "I couldn't do that before—not convincingly."

Kendra had a long road to travel before she reached the right combination of meds that showed her what life could really be like. She tells me about her early teen years, when she struggled with self-harm and suicidal thoughts. Kendra was first put on antidepressants around the age of thirteen and was treated by someone she calls "the worst psychiatrist I've met in my life" (though she said it's a very close call as to which psychiatrist has been the worst to her—there were several). Her medication was changed a handful of times over the course of two years, and following one switch, Kendra attempted suicide. After her mother discovered what had happened, Kendra was rushed to the emergency room, and she had a three-day mandatory stay in the hospital. "During which time," she says, "the psychiatrist didn't return my parents' calls until after I was out of the hospital."

After making a switch to a better psychiatrist, Kendra got to college and eventually swore off both antidepressants and psychiatric care, following what felt like a pointless search for something that might work. "I did muddle through for a couple of years, and there were ups and downs," she says. But the depression and suicidal ideation worsened over time, and Kendra felt compelled to go back to a psychiatrist, which resulted in another failed attempt at antidepressant treatment. "So that was the second time that I swore off psychiatrists and antidepressants," she says.

After starting a doctorate program and facing mounting pressures as a PhD candidate, Kendra once again asked for a referral to a psychiatrist. Her counselor at the time gave her two options—one psychiatrist whose reputation was "okay" and was covered under insurance, or another psychiatrist who had an excellent reputation but who didn't take Kendra's insurance. "And I was like, 'Okay, I'll make it work and go to the one who's really good,' because I could not handle being mistreated by a psychiatrist again," she says. "And he was really good."

The new psychiatrist took time to dig deeper into Kendra's history, which led him to suggest that the diagnosis of depression was probably not accurate for her. "He was the first person who said, 'Maybe it's not just depression; maybe it's bipolar disorder,'" she says. "And the good news is that if you realize it's bipolar disorder and you treat it with the right medicines, you can actually have good results." Kendra was put on a combination of the anti-seizure medication Lamictal and Seroquel, an atypical antipsychotic shown to be effective for bipolar disorder. "That combination of medicines was the first time in my life that I ever just felt stable and okay, and that this must be what just normal people feel like," she says. "And it was absolutely life-changing."

This experience provided Kendra with a baseline of what "stable" might look like in her life. Although she continued to change medications over the years as she and her partner tried to get pregnant and later succeeded, she makes the link between those initial years of stability and a path to a healthier place. "It was like a reset switch of being able to get past the repeating cycles and never being able to dig myself out of it," she says. Without finding that right combination, Kendra doesn't know how her life would have turned out. "I don't know if I would have become stable enough to hold down a job... or have a career." A recent diagnosis of ADHD has also clarified for her the root cause of some of her mental health issues. "It's no longer a mystery of why things have gone the way they have," she says.

I relate a lot to Kendra's experience of finding stable and fulfilling times after taking mental health medications. Drugs have gotten me through very rough patches in my life, and I would go so far as to say that they made me feel like a better person. I was calmer, less likely to have outbursts of anger, and better able to bond with my babies when postpartum anxiety threatened to take my sanity and my ability to mother my children.

But, as with Kendra, it hasn't all been unicorns and rainbows. My first six months on Effexor was a small taste of what life could be like without anxiety and depression, but the effectiveness petered out over time and the side effects became burdensome. After that, I was never able to find a medication that worked over the long term, but I also had no desire to continue trying the many different options. When my love affair with mental health meds cooled, I felt anger and frustration toward both the drug industry and health care providers. Until that point, I'd been sold a rosy picture of "pills for the mind" as a tool to help me not only survive but thrive. And it wasn't only the medical system selling me this vision—I heard positive stories from friends and family members, especially from those for whom medication had been life-changing.

Women navigate a modern mental health system that asks for our faith. We are asked to trust that what is written on the prescription pad, the therapy we are told we need, and the institutions into which we are committed are on our side, designed to fix us up and get us back to our essential roles as caregivers, mothers, and strong and independent working women. As Vigod says, patients often want a perfect treatment, and that doesn't exist in the field of mental health, nor in many other fields of medicine for that matter. For some of us, this has been a hard pill to swallow.

TAKE A CHILL PILL, LADY

IT'S NOT A NEW PHENOMENON for women to be peddled pills for everything that ails them. But contrary to popular perception, the precursors to antidepressants were not developed as part of a conspiracy to get the female population medicated and soothed into domestic complacency. In fact, many drugs have been accidental discoveries, as scientists hunted for cures for other diseases and illnesses. Since the link between these chemicals and improved mood was discovered, the clinical research to study their effectiveness and harms has mostly been in male animals and adult male humans, which means that much of what we know about side effects relates to the male body.

Following the development of mental health medications, women were targeted in advertisements for tranquilizers, sedatives, and antidepressants, which resulted in more frequent prescriptions to women, especially by family doctors.[14] Psychiatrist Jonathan Metzl argues that popular media portrayed patients in need of tranquilizers as "frigid women, wanton women, unmarried women and other women who threatened to keep their wartime jobs, neglect their duties in nuclear households or reject their husbands' amorous advances."[15]

IN THE 1950S, the tranquilizer marketed as Miltown made a huge splash in America and around the world as a drug that could fix any emotional problem, even though the "problems" usually related to a woman's role in the home and wider society. Miltown was not originally developed to be pushed to "hysterical housewives." It was discovered quite by accident when scientist Frank Berger was working on a method of preserving penicillin and stumbled on the discovery that the chemical mephenesin seemed to have a soothing effect on his laboratory animals. Even though sales fell after Miltown was found to be habit-forming (and newer drugs came on the market), the drug's discovery set the stage for an explosion of psychopharmaceuticals that eventually found their way into the medicine cabinets of millions of women worldwide. Metzl proposes that "psychopharmaceuticals came of age in a post-war consumer culture intimately concerned with the role of mothers in maintaining individual and communal peace of mind. As a result, the 1950s set precedents connecting women and psychopharmaceuticals that lay the foundation for 'Mother's Little Helpers' in the decades to come."[16]

If we travel back to the golden age of direct-to-consumer advertising of mood-modifying drugs such as Miltown, we can see a significant increase in the total number of ads over the mid-twentieth century, jumping from just six different ads in 1959 to 247 in 1975.[17] Among these, 40 percent had a woman as the primary figure compared with 30 percent using a man. The ads that depicted female patients were repeated at a higher rate than the ads depicting male patients, and the female characters were portrayed as neurotic, anxious, or a burden on the doctor. The push to get Miltown, and later Valium and Prozac, into the hands of distressed ladies has been big business. Frank Berger later became disillusioned by the way psychiatric drugs were being marketed, and he campaigned against direct-to-consumer advertising.[18] He believed that people should be properly informed about a drug's scientific information rather than manipulated with tactics that appealed to their emotions.

Advertisements from the early 2000s have also been studied, and women were still depicted as the predominant users of antidepressant drugs compared with men, who were the predominant target for cardiovascular drugs. In these ads, men have heart attacks, and women just have depression.[19]

A review of the marketing of prescription drugs in the U.S. found an increase in spending from $17.7 billion in 1997 to $29.9 billion in 2016, with much of this being spent on marketing to health care professionals.[20] While many countries around the world have banned direct-to-consumer advertising (New Zealand and the U.S. still allow it), the marketing that targets health care professionals continues to shape prescription practices.[21] A doctor's choice to prescribe a drug could be influenced by biased medical education, pharmaceutical benefits (such as funds for research, speaker fees, and free samples), and the gender bias that permeates the clinical assessment of women's distress.

Research shows that when a woman presents at her doctor's office with complaints of anxiety or a depressive mood, she is almost twice as likely to be prescribed psychotropic medications compared with men.[22] And this is a practice that has changed over time, with an escalation of prescription patterns for female patients globally. The proposed explanations for these patterns are numerous, and the promotional push from pharmaceutical companies has certainly played a role in the late twentieth and early twenty-first centuries. But there are other factors that might influence prescription practices, including the fact that women are more likely to report their problems and seek help for symptoms compared to men.[23] However, the data showing that women are twice as likely to leave a doctor's office with a prescription can't be fully explained by help-seeking behavior.

In a cross-sectional study from Sweden, researchers found that it was twice as common for women as for men to use antidepressants when they were not currently depressed, as measured by a commonly used depression scale. The authors proposed that one explanation for this might be that these women's depression was in remission at the time, but their findings could also suggest that women are being overtreated with antidepressants. "It seems that even mild symptoms are now considered indicative of disease and treated with medications, although the efficacy is often limited in mild to moderate depression," they write.[24]

IT'S CHEMISTRY, BABY!

PROZAC WAS MARKETED as a "wonder drug" that would fix an apparent serotonin imbalance in the brains of depressed people. It was embraced by more than 33 million Americans in 2002, fourteen years after it was first approved in the U.S.[25] Psychologist Lauren Slater wrote a book about her miraculous transformation on Prozac, from an unemployed and suicidal twentysomething to a professionally successful and happily married woman a decade later.[26] She wasn't alone in her claims that Prozac was life-changing, and many other articles and books painted a similar rosy picture. For people who had struggled with long-term depression, Prozac represented hope and a potential cure.

After the heyday of Prozac, many other SSRIs were approved for use for various mental health disorders, including brand names such as Zoloft, Celexa, Paxil, and Lexapro. Atypical antidepressants don't just work on one neurotransmitter but have multiple ways of acting on the brain, and include Wellbutrin, Remeron, and SNRIs such as Effexor.[27] Much of what I refer to in this section relates to SSRIs, which are the drugs most commonly prescribed to people with depression or anxiety. The premise for the drugs' efficacy is that the depressed brain is lacking in specific neurotransmitters, the primary one being serotonin. As the story goes, serotonin is the wellspring of happy moods, and when we don't have enough of it, we get sad. To fix this "chemical imbalance," we need to pop our daily pill, and presto, we are restored as functioning members of society.

As described earlier in this chapter, neurotransmitters carry messages between cells, attaching themselves to the receptors of the receiving cell. If you understand a bit about American football, think of a sending cell as the quarterback who launches the football (the message) across the line (the synapse). The receiver (the receptor on the end of the receiving cell) catches that football. Once the neurotransmitters have done their job passing their messages to the receptors, they get reabsorbed into the sending cell through the transporter, or "reuptake pump." SSRIs specifically act to prevent the reuptake from happening, which means more of the neurotransmitters hang out in the synapse having a big postgame serotonin bash. There are different types of neurotransmitters, but monoamines (serotonin, dopamine, epinephrine, and several others) include the neurotransmitters that are directly targeted by common antidepressants.[28]

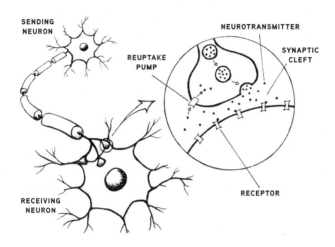

We can't test neurotransmitter levels directly from the human brain or from tissue in our bodies, because that would mean drilling into our skulls and sampling brain tissue (a horrifying image). This means that we rely on animal models for a lot of what we know and understand about neurotransmission and mood. Studies that measure brain serotonin do so in animals such as rats; in humans, studies use a proxy measure of our body's main serotonin metabolite, 5-hydroxyindoleacetic acid (5-HIAA).[29] The ratio of the concentrations of 5-HIAA to serotonin (5-HT) helps researchers to calculate a fairly accurate picture of serotonin neurotransmission. Neuroimaging studies can also provide a picture of the serotonin transporter (which cleans up serotonin from the synapse).

Many neuroscientists and psychiatrists would concede today that the chemical imbalance interpretation of neurotransmitters and mood is oversimplified but not altogether wrong. (A large overview published in 2022 found no consistent relationship between serotonin and depression, and it found some evidence that long-term antidepressant use reduces serotonin concentration.)[30] The brain is complicated, and serotonin is not the only neurotransmitter implicated in mental illness; it's likely that antidepressants are affecting multiple neurotransmitter systems at the same time. Because of the uncertainty surrounding the low serotonin, or chemical imbalance, hypothesis, many people are concerned about the fact that we don't have a clear understanding of how and why antidepressants work on the brain to resolve mood-based symptoms.[31]

"I don't disagree with the chemical imbalance theory, but it's a very vague term," says Jayashri Kulkarni, a professor of psychiatry and director of HER Centre Australia and Monash Alfred Psychiatry Research Centre in Melbourne. In her earlier work with women suffering from schizophrenia, Kulkarni found that an antipsychotic medication used properly worked very well, suggesting that the symptoms got better because of a change in brain chemistry.

"But what we have to understand is, how does this chemical imbalance happen in other conditions?" says Kulkarni. She uses the example of a woman who has experienced incest in her childhood. "We do see that anything like a sexual abuse story in earlier life has such profound changes downstream," she says. The violent household is the social context in which the young girl grew up, and the psychological impact of the abuse results in low self-esteem, "because this woman then grows up to think that she somehow brought this on herself, that she's a bad person, that she does not deserve good things."

Kulkarni explains that there is a layer of biological changes taking place in the brain of the young girl, because of chronic high levels of stress hormones. You may recall from Chapter 3 that chronic stress changes the hypothalamic-pituitary-adrenal axis. "The stress hormones are the messenger systems that impact the neurochemistry systems, which then also impact on the neurocircuitry systems in the brain," says Kulkarni. This may result in a different type of depression that does not respond as well to an antidepressant.

"I think probably what has happened is that there are certain types of depressive illness that are serotonin or noradrenergic, neurochemical based, and they are the ones that respond the best to the SSRI class of drugs, or the SNRI class of drugs," she says. Hormone-based depressions have a different cause and therefore a different mechanism of action within the body and brain.

"Our hypothesis that we're working on, and we're showing some good results, is that trauma- or violence-induced depression is a glutamate system responsive change," says Kulkarni. Glutamate is understood to be one of the most prolific of all neurotransmitters, acting a bit like a giant rave of hopped-up free amino acids in the brain. They have excitatory effects on nerve cells, making them so excited, in fact, that they can usher cells to a swift and untimely death. Either too much glutamate or too little glutamate can be harmful to our brains and bodies.[32]

Kulkarni's work has tested novel and promising treatments to better regulate the glutamate system, including the drug memantine hydrochloride, commonly used to treat symptoms of Alzheimer's disease.[33] Dysfunction in our glutamate system has also been studied in relation to a number of mental health disorders, including bipolar disorder and depression. Single-dose ketamine, a painkiller and anesthetic drug, has also shown some potential as a novel treatment for a glutamate-based mental illness, but results are limited by the low quality of evidence from trials that have been conducted to date.[34] And unfortunately, the side-effect profile of ketamine can be just as troublesome as that of an SSRI.

Until newer drugs are proven clinically effective, cost-effective, and safe for widespread use, antidepressants will remain the go-to for most clinicians. "I think the mainstream drugs are splashed around far too readily," says Kulkarni. "Oncologists have a wide array of cancer drugs, but they also have the markers for the cells, so you can match one to the other." What she means is that physicians can provide more targeted treatment for different types of cancer, matching drugs to the tumor or stage of disease. The lack of biomarkers in psychiatry means clinicians must make an educated guess, and if that guess is wrong, the consequences for patients can be significant.

ADVENTURES IN SIDE EFFECTS

AFTER SEVERAL MONTHS on Effexor, I started to notice strange side effects. Before meds, I would cry at the drop of a hat, but on meds, I was as cool as a cucumber. I didn't shed a tear when my grandfather was diagnosed with advanced cancer and passed away weeks later; it felt as though I was an objective observer of his illness and death. This was slightly awkward given how devastated the rest of my family felt. When I weaned off the medication some months later, I experienced a delayed grief that I had been unable to process on the drug.

My body began twitching involuntarily. I noticed this while working at the computer: my leg would jerk to one side, or my hand would move the mouse an inch. Though my anxiety over food and my body image waned, I lost a ton of weight without even trying. My libido also tanked, a side effect that, unexpectedly, seems to affect men more than women.[35] And then the medication just stopped working. After about a year, I noticed that the positive effects were wearing off and my anxiety was creeping back.

That antidepressants can lose effectiveness over time (amusingly called the "poop-out effect") or after repeated treatments is something that patients have drawn attention to, but the lack of medical knowledge as to why this happens can be frustrating for those of us who feel like we're acting as guinea pigs for a range of mental health medications. Theories have been proposed but not proven. For example, it may be that since our body works to maintain homeostasis (a physiological balance of the body), it brings serotonin levels back down after the drug initially increases them. Another possible explanation is that adaptations in other neurotransmitter systems (such as norepinephrine) may contribute to the loss in effectiveness.[36]

Writer and artist Julie Green shares a similar experience to mine: initially, she found that Celexa (the brand name for the ssri citalopram) was a magic bullet. As she writes in an article for *Chatelaine*, the drug "worked wonders for me—until it didn't."[37] Julie told me later that she had been prescribed an antidepressant for a short period in her twenties, but after a bout of postpartum depression following the birth of her son, her doctor recommended she stay on the drug for the long term. "My doctor said...'You have to be on the drug because it could happen again and you need to be stable. You're a mom.'"

Julie went along with her doctor's advice until her son was approaching his tween years and she seemed to hit a therapeutic wall. "I felt like my depression was coming back a bit, but I also just felt quite numb," says Julie. "I didn't feel anything—I didn't really feel like myself." She had been dealing with side effects as well, such as loss of libido, weight gain, sleep issues, and suicidality, which seemed to increase in intensity the longer she stayed on the drug. "It wasn't working, and it may have ultimately been making things worse."

Side effects for antidepressant medications are common across the sexes, and there is still no clear consensus on whether there are sex-related (or biological) differences in the drugs' effectiveness. Some studies have shown that females respond better to antidepressants, while others show that males respond better than females.[38] What we do know is that there are sex differences in pharmacokinetics, which is the study of how a drug is absorbed, distributed, metabolized, and eliminated from our bodies. The pharmacokinetics in females is telling, and a study conducted by Irving Zucker and Brian Prendergast describes the impact: "Among patients administered a standard drug dose, females are exposed to higher blood drug concentrations and longer drug elimination times than males. This likely contributes to the near doubling of adverse drug reactions in female patients, raising the possibility that women are routinely overmedicated."[39] ("Overmedicated" in the sense that the drug's dosage may be too high in some cases, not in the sense that it should never have been prescribed in the first place.)

The limited data we have tells us that women are more likely to experience allostatic load (physiological stress on the body) when taking antidepressants compared with men.[40] This leads to a disruption in our metabolic, immune, neuroendocrine, and cardiovascular systems. When challenges such as racism, poverty, inequality, and violence or trauma start to pile up (in other words, chronic stress), our physiological systems become overloaded. Exactly how antidepressant medication seems to impact that load is still up for debate, but it could relate back to the theory that our bodies are constantly trying to maintain our physiological equilibrium. When antidepressants disrupt that equilibrium, some women may experience worsening allostatic load, potentially leading to poorer mental health outcomes.

Given the systemic underrepresentation of women in clinical trials, and the fact that most studies do not test drugs at different stages in the menstrual cycle,[41] we don't know enough about why the drugs' side effects are more burdensome on female bodies. Adverse drug reactions have been observed for antipsychotics, TCAs, atypical antidepressants, SNRIs, and SSRIs, and sex differences in drug pharmacokinetics have been linked to sex differences in adverse drug reactions. The long list of adverse reactions in females includes things like severe weight gain, type 2 diabetes, tremor, suicidal ideation, dry mouth, dizziness, and delusions.[42] There is some evidence from patients that certain side effects are only associated with long-term use of antidepressants.[43]

Part of the problem might be that most drugs are prescribed to women and men at the same doses and in the same form. "Depending on the properties of the medication, people who are female might sometimes benefit from lower doses of a drug, or longer intervals between doses for injectables," says Simone Vigod. Her work centers on the perinatal period, about which there is even less research to inform patients and clinicians about medication use. "Most medications were not tested in women, never mind pregnant people," says Vigod. "We haven't considered sex and gender properly, even in the development and making of doses and thinking about side effects of these medications."

Within-female differences (meaning differences that occur between one group of women and another group, rather than in women compared to men) are also important to understand. Concerns about this have been raised for other prescriptions, like hormonal birth control, which comes in standardized doses.[44] Within groups of women and between individuals, we may see different responses and different adverse effects based on our unique biopsychosocial factors.

WHEN I STARTED NOTICING the worsening side effects from Effexor, I paid a visit to my doctor—and the response was not encouraging. Many other women have told me similar stories. Women who report side effects to their physicians may be dismissed or told that the effects are unrelated to the prescribed drug. Doctors might also switch a patient to an alternative drug, add another drug (such as an anti-psychotic), or adjust the dose.[45] "I'm sick of seeing women who have been prescribed antipsychotics, for no apparent reason," says Kulkarni of this practice. "Why is this woman who's never had a psychotic symptom in her life on this big dose, which has got all these side effects?"

Adding another drug to treat side effects from the first drug is called a "prescribing cascade." Clinicians often mis-interpret the side effect for a new medical condition.[46] Out of nine common prescribing cascades that have been observed to affect older people (older women especially), four involve psychotropic medications like antipsychotics, benzodiaz-epines, and ssris or snris.[47] All of these drugs are being added on because the doctor believes that the new symptom is evidence of another problem.

What doesn't seem to be happening is an open discus-sion about whether the woman should continue to take the original drug. In Julie's case, when she brought her list of concerns about Celexa to her doctor, she was advised not to go off the medication. "Her concern was always being stable for my son," says Julie, whose child was diagnosed with autism in early childhood. And so she remained on the drug for many years. "I took her advice and stayed on it, because she said, 'Look, you're just going to keep relapsing. Basically, this is just how it is for some people genetically.'"

A notion central to the feminist critique of the way that depressed women are medicated is that it serves to help her function properly in her feminine role and uphold her "service" to society and her family.[48] If our depression arises partly from experiences like sexual harassment and violence, trauma, the mental load from care work, marginalization, devaluation, and poverty, it's a curious thing that our society focuses almost solely on a chemical fix for a problem not created by us, but affecting us. To remain dedicated mothers, engaged citizens, or professional go-getters, we receive the message to just take our meds and get on with things.

PRECISION MEDICINE AND THE FUTURE OF MENTAL HEALTH MEDS

HUMOR ME FOR A MOMENT and join me on a journey through the ideal mental health system in our modern world. Let's assume that a young woman is experiencing anxiety and depression for the first time in her life.

The stigma and shame have lifted, and she finds it easy to talk to friends, family, and teachers about the symptoms she's experiencing. This open dialogue directs her to online resources, where she reads more about mental health and the experiences of different people from around the world. When she visits her family doctor, they don't seem frustrated with her or surprised by her condition, because training and experience have prepared them for what they need to do to help. First, they talk about the severity of her symptoms, to determine whether her anxiety and depression require medical treatment or could be solved with both individual and community-based solutions. She is screened for a history of trauma and asked whether she is currently facing any threat of physical or sexual violence. She feels that her symptoms are worsening, and she cannot pinpoint any situational cause that would have triggered the illness.

There are options for medical tests that lead to a reliable diagnosis and a range of treatment options. When the results are in, she and her doctor sit together and go over the options, and that process helps her to assess her own values and preferences. She decides that a combination of therapy, social support, and medication feels like the best fit. The medications available are numerous, but based on her personal genetic profile and symptoms, they choose a medication likely to suit her. At this point, they discuss medication withdrawal—what she can expect when she chooses to come off the drug. Her doctor schedules a follow-up appointment in four weeks but tells her to call the office if she's experiencing difficult side effects or if her symptoms are worsening. She is also provided with guidelines for the length of treatment with medication, suggesting that they begin with six months and reassess as they go. She is referred to a culturally competent therapist covered under the country's universal health care plan and meets with a community liaison to access nonmedical supports in her neighborhood.

One year later, she is feeling much better and chooses to come off the medication. Her doctor supports her decision and provides her with very clear guidelines for a slow withdrawal and tips for coping with the side effects of discontinuation. She is warned that symptoms will worsen for a period, and she is given a sick note for paid time off work as she goes through the worst of the withdrawal. After six months, she is feeling back to herself, and life goes on.

"PSYCHIATRY IS VERY PRIMITIVE," says Jayashri Kulkarni. "We don't actually have the objective biomarkers yet to clearly say, 'This is what's going on.'" Kulkarni feels frustrated that psychiatry is unlike cardiology and oncology (for example), where there are more accurate diagnostic markers and treatment options that have proven to be effective. "We need the ECG for the mind," she says. An electrocardiogram determines how well your heart is functioning by measuring its electrical activity.

"When you take a psychiatric drug, you do so on faith," writes Lauren Slater in her book documenting her thirty-five years of experience with psychotropic drugs. "The truth is that while we have dozens and dozens of psychiatric drugs ... we still have no actual blood or urine or tissue test with which to determine the particular psychiatric illness a person suffers from."[49] This is precisely why the "You'd take insulin if you had diabetes" platitudes don't sit well with some of us, because diabetes can be clearly diagnosed and the drug measurably acts to fix what is dysfunctional in the body.

"The problem is that an SSRI is a bit like taking paracetamol [acetaminophen] for a fever," says Kulkarni. "You know you'll bring the fever down, but you don't really know what you're treating. You could be treating malaria, you could be treating the flu, you could be treating some weird drug reaction." Antidepressants may make a dent in our sadness, lethargy, or hopelessness, but they can't always tackle the source of the problem. Kulkarni's research work has focused mainly on the social and psychological sides of treatment in addition to the biological, so that a woman's social situation is being addressed and therapy is helping her to tackle some of the psychological impacts to make daily living easier.

"At the same time, psychiatrists' personal biases also play a part because we're the tool that's actually trying to understand this individual's contextual issues, social life, as well as psychological makeup and any biological changes that are going on," she says. "Let's use drugs sensibly and try and target symptoms more accurately involving more precise medicine."

Less than 20 percent of health care professionals routinely use rating scales or other clinical tools for diagnosing and monitoring mental health symptoms, whereas they use measurement tools for other physical symptoms in their daily practice.[50] In many trials, measurement-based care outperforms routine care (or "care as usual"), which uses clinical knowledge, past experience, and gut instinct (all of which, as I've argued, are subject to bias). If I see my family doctor for routine blood work, various markers, such as low-density lipoprotein (LDL) are monitored, especially if I have genetic or other disease risk factors. At a certain LDL cutoff point, I would be diagnosed with high cholesterol, and my doctor would provide specific guidelines to help me lower my cholesterol, whether through lifestyle changes or medication.

In the ideal scenario I created above, genetic tests help to streamline diagnosis and treatment. Research suggests that over 50 percent of the variance of antidepressant response and tolerability is genetically controlled. However, very few genetic (and nongenetic) biomarkers have been fully studied and implemented in practice.[51] Precision psychiatry aims to make use of available genetic tests and to integrate the psychosocial aspects of a person's mental health to personalize treatment—which is essential, because environmental factors can affect gene expression.[52]

Kulkarni wants to see more of this being developed and tested within psychiatry, so that there are objective diagnostic markers. Without them, she says, "we're leaving the field open to subjective diagnoses and subjective treatments, and that has led to a whole range of odd practices." The people on the receiving end of these odd practices are the patients, who can sometimes experience harm and poor outcomes.

It is worth noting that, as I proposed in earlier chapters, we may need to accept a certain level of uncertainty in mental illness. If the mind and personal experience are affected by our social world as much as we think they are, then it's possible that no diagnostic test could ever paint the full picture. But getting to some level of precision when it comes to medication would hopefully be an improvement on the "spray and pray" method we have now, where it's anyone's guess as to which drug might work.

New genetic tests are showing some early promise in predicting antidepressant treatment response and remission rates, although evidence is limited and many trials are industry-sponsored, which can add significant bias to the methods and findings.[53] The other issue with genetic testing is the cost. In Canada, where I live, one Health Technology Assessment (HTA) study estimated a multimillion-dollar price tag for adding these tests to our health care budget.[54] Yet this same assessment found that people suffering from depression and their caregivers supported genetic testing, because they saw its potential to help them receive effective treatment, to minimize side effects, and to avoid the trial-and-error issue of psychotropic medications.

Despite the lack of clarity on the benefits of genetic testing in the treatment of mental illness, there is something to be said for defining what *type* of mental health disorder women are suffering from, by digging deeper than the standard depression symptom checklist. Kulkarni identifies different types of depression, based on factors such as hormonal changes or a history of trauma, which would impact the stress response system and thereby change brain chemistry over the long term. Other researchers have studied blood tests that could identify whether a person was experiencing a depression associated with inflammation in the body. One study found that when patients had high levels of inflammation at the beginning of the trial, they experienced lower depression severity when treated with a combined bupropion-SSRI versus an SSRI alone.[55] Bupropion (Wellbutrin) is an atypical antidepressant that can act as an anti-inflammatory, lowering levels of a biomarker that can be measured by a blood test.

The EMBARC study at the University of Texas Southwestern Medical Center examined clinical and biological markers to predict different treatment outcomes with a two-phase clinical trial: the first phase studied sertraline (Zoloft) versus a placebo, and the second phase studied sertraline versus bupropion.[56] What's unique about this study is that clinical markers were taken into consideration: whether someone was "anxious depressed," their gender, and whether they'd experienced trauma, as well as markers that looked more closely at subtypes of depression (for instance, atypical depression, a label women often receive, which is linked to anxiety symptoms, suicidal behavior, longer episodes, and a periodic reversal in symptoms—where people "perk up" when something positive happens).[57]

Taken together, these promising advancements provide hope for those of us for whom mental health meds have not been the "happy pill" we once hoped they'd be. Until the day these tools are widely available and effective, personalized medicine in mental health care needs to focus on patient-centered care, a better understanding of women's personal situations, and individual values and preferences.

IT'S DIFFICULT TO WRITE or talk about medication use for mental illness without falling into one of two traps: the first is to propose that medication is an evil invention of Big Pharma, and it at best works no better than a placebo and at worst is very harmful; the other is to insist that medication is the only way to correct mental illness, and everyone should be on it. In writing this chapter, I did a quick search on Instagram and came up with thirty thousand posts with the hashtag #TakeYourMeds, with encouraging and positive messages about the benefits of mental health meds. Meanwhile, on Twitter and other platforms, there are hundreds of accounts that are openly anti-medication or anti-psychiatry and make dubious claims about the drugs' inefficacy. Then there are those of us caught in the middle, making tough decisions about medication use, which is a personal choice that involves our values and preferences and an accounting of the benefits and risks—hopefully in collaboration with a trusted health care provider.

When making these complex decisions, it really comes down to trusting ourselves and listening to our bodies. I learned how to listen to my body and knew deep down that SSRIS were not the right choice for me, but it took years of turmoil and stress to come to that realization. If I had been guided by health professionals, perhaps with a tool like a patient decision aid, I know I would have saved myself a lot of grief. My wish is for *all* women to have access to effective biopsychosocial treatment options, to consent only once properly informed, to receive support for their preferences and values, and to have better care in coming off medication. This can be done in collaboration with psychiatrists, psychologists, social workers, patient advocates, and anyone else working toward better mental health care. In other words, we can find common ground to stand on, a place where the door opens to choices for each and every individual who wants them.

10

MAKING PEACE
WITH OUR MOODS

> We can endure almost any pain if we can hope
> that it will pass. But when we are convinced that
> it will never pass, it is unbearable.
>
> **LUCY MAUD MONTGOMERY**[1]

IN HIGH SCHOOL, my best friend and I were obsessed with the *Anne of Green Gables* television series created by Kevin Sullivan (not to be confused with *Anne With an E*, the reboot that streams on Netflix). We watched those DVDs on repeat, eating copious snacks and sniffling our way through the scene of Matthew's death. I had read all the Anne books in my childhood and felt a close kinship with the redheaded orphan—not because I'd had a similar childhood experience, but because I admired the way she wore her emotions on her sleeve with wild abandon. Sadness was "the depths of despair," and happiness was "a new day, with no mistakes in it." As a child who felt everything from the darkest depths to the wildest of joys, I felt Anne gave me permission to be my wonderful and weird self, and in her I found the hope of embracing the person I was and not the person I thought I ought to be. "There's such a lot of different Annes in me," says Anne. "I sometimes think that is why I'm such a troublesome person. If I was just the one Anne, it would be ever so much more comfortable, but then it wouldn't be half so interesting."

It didn't surprise me, then, to later learn that the author who imagined such a daring and feisty character had herself faced the darkness of mental illness.[2] It is palpable in the way that she takes the reader into the storm of Anne's struggles and emotions, the exasperation of those who endure her wild mood swings, and the ways in which Anne matures into adulthood and struggles against those versions of herself. Lucy Maud Montgomery's fictional tales and her personal diaries are full of references to hope: that most elusive of emotions that emboldens us to trudge our way through pain, not necessarily because there is a promise of a reward at the end of it all, but simply because we recognize that when something passes (as it's always apt to do), something new arises. Hope is a recognition of transience and transformation.

To find a path toward healing, I had to learn two things: the first is that I am not broken; the second is that my emotional pain will pass, that it is something I can endure—and perhaps even welcome into my life. I don't want to argue that suffering is something we should all be accepting with open arms, because in our modern Western society especially, we tend to turn our backs on those who carry the heaviest burdens. Suggesting that someone should just "accept" suffering is dismissive and doesn't address the social and structural challenges that contribute to high rates of mental illness.

For myself, though, there was value in understanding that (at the risk of being overly simplistic) life is hard and scary. There is no cure for that. My earlier understanding of my mental illness was that there was an answer I was seeking, and once I found "the thing" (be it medication, therapy, or alternatives like the ones I'll cover in the next chapter) everything would fall into place. Instead, I have learned to sit with pain in the deepest darkness of my mind and body and ride the waves without knowing when the next wave might come and overwhelm me. But I also learned a little secret along the way, that no one had ever told me: with each new threatening emotion, each relapse into anxiety and depression, it became easier to ride the waves.

My unlearning began after I had my second child and decided to wean off my meds for the fourth and final time. Medication had served me well in times of crisis, and I'm grateful it will be there for me in the future, should I ever need it again. But I realized that over the long term, medication was not an effective tool for me; it was like trying to hammer a nail using a screwdriver. Medication helped level the playing field of my emotions, but it left me with an empty, stagnant feeling that I could not get past, and a mountain of side effects that I was no longer willing to accept.

This process of unlearning can happen whether you are medicated or not. For some people, medication is the gate through which we walk toward healthier coping strategies, and it can be a much-needed alternative to the problematic self-medicating we sometimes do with food, recreational drugs, or alcohol. Medication can make all the difference in an individual's ability to feel their emotions, to gain strength, and to be able to participate in therapy that addresses the biopsychosocial elements of their distress.

The things I share in this chapter cannot (and should not) apply to everyone and are not a remedy for your own personal pain. But I hope they provide you with a new and refreshing frame of reference, and maybe a sense of hope. Making peace with my moods meant that I had to wrestle with who I was as a "self," and all the ways in which the biological, psychological, and social elements of my selfhood converged. Once medication was out of my life, I knew it was imperative that I build a strong network of social support and individual self-care practices that I could lean on when things got rough. I was on the hunt for tools that could help me dive down to the bottom of my pain and then learn how to swim back up to the surface.

But first I had to successfully come off my medication, and that proved to be a way bigger challenge than I had anticipated.

STOP THE TRAIN: COPING WITH ANTIDEPRESSANT WITHDRAWAL

BY THE TIME my second daughter turned one, I wasn't in any hurry to come off my medication. It seemed to lessen the intensity of my symptoms, and I was worried about relapsing. My doctor continued to prescribe me refills, and there was no discussion about whether I should consider alternatives. I was a busy mother and had little time for self-care. I did find a private therapist who allowed me to bring my baby to appointments, and a stable job meant I had benefits that would cover five hundred dollars in fees for psychological services per year. That amounted to a total of 3.6 appointments, which was like applying a child-sized bandage to a large gaping wound—but it was still much more than many people have. My husband and I decided we would pay for additional therapy out of pocket so that I could receive adequate care.

As time passed and my baby turned into a toddler, the side effects of the medication started to increase in number and severity. My libido tanked, but it was less severe than when I was taking Effexor. The twitching was noticeably better, or maybe it was the fact that I was distracted with two young children. After eighteen months on the medication, I began to experience intense heartburn, usually when I was eating a late dinner or hadn't eaten for a long time. And this wasn't the kind of heartburn that could be relieved with a couple of Tums; it was overwhelming pain that radiated from my stomach all the way up to my throat. I also had episodes of vertigo, which would lay me out flat for a full day. Lifting my head off the floor was enough to send me spiraling into dizziness and nausea, and I couldn't physically care for my children. It's possible that the medication and these symptoms weren't linked, but I haven't experienced them since going off the medication.

The drug's effectiveness also wore off over time, and I didn't want to risk bumping up my dose and potentially experiencing worsening side effects. My doctor was understandably concerned that I wanted to come off antidepressants, given the research showing that repeated relapses may signal the need for an individual to stay on medication long term (meaning forever).[3] Some people do need to stay on antidepressants to prevent a recurrence of their mental illness, but research shows that in 30 to 50 percent of users, there is no evidence indicating that they should continue their medication once symptoms have resolved.[4]

There are no clear guidelines for maintenance treatment with antidepressants for depression or anxiety. Much of what's available was published before 2013 and generally recommends that treatment last between six and twelve months, with patients at risk of a depression relapse sometimes being told to remain on the medication forever.[5] The Royal College of Psychiatrists in the U.K. updated their guidelines in 2019 to recommend a minimum of six months' treatment with antidepressants after "full symptom remission" and for people with a history of recurrent depression to continue on for at least two years.[6] They do acknowledge that some patients are prescribed antidepressants for much longer than two years.

There was little guidance available to my doctor on how I should stop the medication, other than recommendations for slow tapering over several weeks. The National Institute for Health and Care Excellence (NICE) updated its guidelines in 2022 for the treatment of depression and recommends that people talk to the person who first prescribed their medication (usually a GP or other mental health professional). The guidelines state that "it is usually necessary to reduce the dose in stages over time (called 'tapering')" and that most people can stop antidepressants successfully.[7]

My doctor wrote me a prescription for half-dose pills, so that I could pop a twenty-five-milligram dose instead of the full fifty, which is the lowest therapeutic dose available for sertraline. I decided to take matters into my own hands, a strategy I had used previously to wean myself off antidepressants. I opened my pills and siphoned off tiny amounts of the drug each day. This was far from a precise method of withdrawal, but it was the only strategy I felt might be effective to prevent some of the more severe withdrawal symptoms I'd experienced in the past.

I took four months to taper off the medication, and after I'd put the final dose on my tongue and swallowed, I was convinced that I had beaten the system. This was the trick that mental health professionals were missing, and I had discovered it by taking medical care into my own hands. I was going to advertise my magical Antidepressant Withdrawal Plan to the masses and transform mental health care!

The following morning, I felt the first of the brain zaps: a zing of electric energy that blurred my vision and made me feel as though I'd walked through an invisible force field. With each zap, my body gave a jolt, and I'd shake off the dizziness until the next one. Soon they came in waves, and I rode each shock with increasing alarm. I started to feel nauseous, and my muscles ached as though I were suffering from the flu. My foolproof plan for antidepressant withdrawal was a sham.

In the coming weeks, I battled through the brain zaps, nausea, mounting depression, and flu-like symptoms, all while parenting two children and working full-time. As summer sun turned to cloudy fall days, I felt my mood worsening.

EARLY TRIALS OF SSRIS found that withdrawal symptoms were mild, not very common, and tended to last only several weeks. Since this time, little research has been done to track patients' withdrawal symptoms, especially after long-term use. A systematic review that explored interventions that are effective in managing antidepressant discontinuation found only two trials that reported on withdrawal symptoms.[8] This is an alarming gap in our scientific knowledge, especially in light of a patient survey that found more than half of respondents experience withdrawal symptoms, and one-quarter report the symptoms as severe.[9]

Another systematic review exploring the incidence, severity, and duration of antidepressant withdrawal found similar outcomes.[10] In this review, almost half of those discontinuing their meds had severe symptoms. Many other studies have since reported data that directly contradicts the initial claim by medical experts that SSRI withdrawal symptoms are usually mild and short in duration. It must be noted that most of this data is survey-based, and surveys are notoriously biased. However, patient stories and patient perspectives matter, and there is mounting anecdotal evidence that for some people, antidepressant withdrawal is not only tough but sometimes impossible.

With changes in prescription practices and more of us staying on antidepressants for long periods of time, it's likely that a significant number of patients will require support if they eventually wish to stop taking medication. Yet few countries have given any time or attention to the problems that patients face when coming off antidepressants. In Canada and the U.S., I couldn't find any trials or ongoing research addressing antidepressant withdrawal practices.

The U.K. is one of the only regions that has seen a big push for research in this area, likely because of the anecdotal evidence of challenging drug withdrawal symptoms that patients and care providers have shared.[11] In 2017, two petitions to parliamentary committees in Scotland and Wales invited participants to submit their experiences with drug withdrawal symptoms, which were then compiled and shared with policymakers.

Studies show that only one in fourteen patients taking long-term antidepressant medication is able to successfully stop.[12] In 2018, the *New York Times* drew attention to the problem with a feature titled "Many people taking antidepressants discover they cannot quit."[13] Anthony Kendrick, a professor of primary care at the University of Southampton in the U.K., is quoted as saying, "Some people are essentially being parked on these drugs for convenience's sake because it's difficult to tackle the issue of taking them off." Kendrick is lead investigator of a large trial called REDUCE, which aims to identify effective, safe, and affordable ways to help patients taper off long-term antidepressant treatment. They are developing and testing an internet-based intervention using CBT methods to support tapering and cessation, and the results will be available after this book is published.

MY JOURNEY DOWN the rabbit hole of research and online discourse about antidepressants showed that both the supporting and dissenting sides were dominated by the voices of men—in academic journals, online editorials, commentaries, and blog posts. The voices of women were difficult to find, unless I scoured online forums or Facebook groups. As I searched for peers who were going through a similar experience to mine, I stumbled across the work of mental health advocate, author, and award-winning chef Brooke Siem, who chronicles her withdrawal journey in a gripping memoir called *May Cause Side Effects*.[14]

"There was not a point from age fifteen to thirty in which I was not medicated up to my eyeballs," says Brooke. She began taking multiple prescription medications as a young teen, including antidepressants to treat her grief after the sudden death of her father, as well as meds for low thyroid, bile reflux disease, acne, and the birth control pill for menstrual pain. "There was never any question about whether or not I should continue to be on the drugs," she says. "No one ever looked at the length of time or the amount of drugs I was on and was like, 'This is a little high, maybe we should adjust this.'" Instead, the refills continued for the next fifteen years.

At the age of thirty, Brooke found herself in a worse place than she'd ever been before, contemplating suicide and struggling to get through each day. One day, she says, she had a lightbulb moment: "I was like, you know, if all these antidepressants were working, maybe I wouldn't be suicidal." The side effects had also become a significant problem, and Brooke noticed difficulties with her short-term memory and cognitive functioning.

Brooke saw a psychiatrist for guidance on getting off the drugs safely, but she faced a lot of opposition. "The psychiatrist was not supportive of my decision to get off these drugs; she was brash, she was dismissive . . . every stereotype a bad psychiatrist can be," says Brooke. The doctor pushed for a switch to another antidepressant. Brooke persisted, and the psychiatrist finally conceded, advising her to go off Effexor cold turkey and telling her that she'd feel like she had the flu for a couple of days. Brooke was likely given this advice because she was already on the lowest prescription dose offered, which meant there wasn't a prescribed option to taper any lower.

"By the time I got through the Effexor withdrawal, because I started that first, the really intense, unbearable part of the withdrawal effects had passed," she says. Then she decided to quit the second antidepressant she was taking. "I got to the Wellbutrin, and I was just so mad at [the psychiatrist] and at the whole situation that I was like, 'I'm getting off this Wellbutrin and I will deal with whatever happens.'"

Just as people can face stigma and shame for choosing to go on medication for mental illness, they can also face stigma and shame for choosing to go off medication. Coming off meds is often subtly or overtly discouraged by well-meaning friends, family, and mental health professionals, and there is contentious discourse about the suggestion that antidepressants may not be effective for everyone, or that withdrawal is difficult. This is understandable given that there are still populations who are underserved and undertreated, but it doesn't help people like Brooke who prefer to come off medication and want to do it safely and effectively.

Brooke's withdrawal experience was a very difficult one, but she didn't have faith in her psychiatrist and didn't feel she could trust or confide in her. "I was having homicidal visions as I was walking down the street, and I was afraid that I was going to hurt myself or somebody else," she says. "I didn't trust that I could tell the psychiatrist that and not have her put me on an involuntary psychiatric hold."

Instead, Brooke called a family friend who happens to be a psychologist. She relayed the scary thoughts she was having and was reassured that what she was experiencing was due to intense withdrawal symptoms. "She pretty much assured me that this was withdrawal, that I wasn't actually crazy, and that I wasn't going to hurt anyone," she says. "And that helped me, you know, turn the heat down on my kettle enough to push through it."

Given that the decision to wean is almost always initiated by the patient, many individuals do not feel that they are properly supported by their medical care providers. Patients often receive significant misinformation and are offered little to no guidance about the best way to taper drugs. Caregivers sometimes dismiss common symptoms, downplay the intensity of those symptoms, or even suggest to patients that they are experiencing a relapse of their mental illness rather than withdrawal.

There is very little knowledge about the differences or similarities between withdrawal symptoms and relapse. My anxiety and depression always came back with a vengeance each time I discontinued my meds, and my doctor and I assumed it was because I was relapsing. I would then go back on the medication and start the whole process all over again. It was a difficult cycle to break. Because of the lack of support and information, most people turn to the internet and social media to fill the void left by health services, and it seems that the majority who do so are women.

An analysis of Facebook support groups for antidepressant withdrawal looked at sixteen groups, with over sixty thousand group members. It found that group membership was 82.5 percent women, and group administrators and moderators were 80 percent women.[15] The members came from many countries, but the majority (over 50 percent) were from the U.S. All the groups were relatively new, having formed on average six years prior to the study (published in 2021). Where the groups' mission statements were available, the authors of the study noted very strong language used in the description of the groups' purpose and goals, including words like "hate," "toxic," or "danger/dangerous." I perused several mission statements myself and observed a strong stance being taken against the use of medication and psychiatry in the treatment of mental illness.

The most common reason for people to seek out Facebook peer groups was a failed doctor- or psychiatrist-led tapering process. Due to short tapering periods (over days or weeks), many patients had experienced serious distress, "followed by a complete loss of belief and faith in the ability of their clinician to support them to safely taper."[16] Most groups posted an alternative tapering schedule, reducing by 10 percent of the previous dose per month, based on older protocols for patients withdrawing from psychiatric drugs such as benzodiazepines.

Peer support groups can be a beneficial and effective intervention for individuals struggling with mental illness, especially when they are delivered online.[17] However, when peer-led groups form out of a failure or a gap in health services, clinicians should be sitting up and asking themselves, What's pushing patients away? In this case, it's a personal health crisis that's being dismissed or minimized by the medical community. If the information given to a person by their family doctor doesn't jibe with that person's lived experience, they will naturally seek out the help they need elsewhere. And it appears that the peer-led supports that have materialized in the place of clinical care can undermine the important work that psychiatrists do, as well as the potential benefits medication can have for many individuals. When I put out a call on Twitter asking for people's peer support tips for weaning from antidepressants, I received a barrage of suggestions for questionable "treatments" like vitamin supplements and other commercial "withdrawal kits." While I've never shied away from trying alternative treatments that have few harms (but maybe little benefit), it's alarming to see what has filled the void created by the medical community's failure to provide patients with good, evidence-based care.

PLANNING FOR SETBACKS

HAVING BEEN ON ANTIDEPRESSANTS for so long, Brooke points out that she had "no baseline to go back to. My only frame of reference for who I was, was as a nonmedicated child." After coming off her meds, Brooke felt like everything she knew about herself had changed; music she'd once enjoyed sounded jarring, and even her taste in food changed. "What the withdrawal process can do is really shine a magnifying glass on things that were already there, because not only are you more primed to notice and feel the terribleness of everything, but you've also been shrouded in this armor for however long," says Brooke. She's referring to the blunting of emotions that some people experience on SSRIs and how intense and overwhelming those emotions can be after they stop taking their meds.

It took almost a year for Brooke to feel confident that she was through the worst of the withdrawal. I ask her how she navigated the withdrawal and managed the setbacks. "Once I started to really trust that when the [emotional] waves came, I would be able to come out of them, I think the real healing started," she says. "I don't think it was any real magic." She also feels that having very clear life and work goals at the time propelled her to accept that she had to just push through. A short time after withdrawing from both antidepressants, Brooke was set to pack her bags and board a one-way flight to Malaysia to travel the world for a year. "I realize this is not the case for everyone ... and I was not looking to have an *Eat, Pray, Love* experience," she says. "I just needed to get on a plane and have my life be different."

I'M A VEGETABLE GARDENER. I don't have much time for shrubs or flowers, but if I can eat it, I will try to grow it. I spend the first half of the year, when my garden is buried under a mountain of snow, planning which vegetables I will grow and purchasing seeds. In March, as the migratory birds are making their way back north, I coax tiny seeds into seedlings, which are delicate creatures. They need hours of strong light, just the right amount of water, and appropriate soil. When it's time to plant my garden, I must wait for the right moment (not too hot, not too cold), and heaven help those poor babies if I plunk them into the ground without first hardening them off—a method by which you introduce your seedlings to the outside world for increasing increments of time, hurrying them back inside if it's too windy or hot.

I realized that my brain after antidepressant withdrawal was like a tiny seedling. The slow and steady tapering meant that I didn't shock my system, but like in gardening, even hardy seedlings must adjust to the outside world. I came to accept that the symptoms I experienced after I finished my last pill were a normal part of the process. To mitigate these symptoms, I took sick days when I needed to rest, worked with a therapist, and tended to the garden of my mind.

The period of withdrawal for some people can be quite long; anecdotal evidence from patients shows that the post-meds period can last for months, rather than weeks.[18] Planning and preparing for a longer time frame of recovery can help you to set realistic expectations (and bonus if you are someone who only has mild symptoms for a few weeks).

Research has highlighted three facilitating factors that help patients discontinue their antidepressant medication:

1. Confidence in your ability to stop;

2. Effective coping strategies; and

3. Stable life circumstances.[19]

Problematic experiences with discontinuing antidepressants and psychological or physical dependence were the two main reasons patients found it hard to stop taking medication. The idea that mental illness is caused by a chemical imbalance also contributed to the patient's belief that it was necessary for them to continue taking antidepressants.

At the time I withdrew from meds, I was partnered, I had friends and family who cared about my well-being, and I was financially able to invest in my own recovery. Withdrawal becomes difficult or near impossible when social and financial supports are not in place, which is something the medical community hasn't even begun to address. At this point in the game, we don't even have proper interventions to support patients who are willing, able, and resourced enough to come off medication.

Researchers from King's College London are testing an online intervention for antidepressant withdrawal that targets general practitioners in the U.K. primary care sector. Family doctors are randomized into two groups: treatment as usual (which means they give whatever advice they would normally give patients attempting to discontinue antidepressant medication) or a computerized decision-support tool to assist with patient decision-making.[20] Much more of this work needs to be done around the world, and it needs to be culturally appropriate. Not all populations will respond well to standardized decision aids or CBT interventions, and social supports like paid sick days need to be in place for individuals who are dealing with more intense side effects.

With my four experiences of tapering off antidepressants, I've come to recognize that some of my mental illness relapse or recurrence was either fully or partially attributable to withdrawal symptoms. It was also sometimes related to specific life situations, like pregnancy and postpartum. I've developed the skills that allow me to clearly see the difference between "I'm depressed for a very good reason" and "I'm a mess and I have no idea why or how to get through this." Developing these skills didn't make me *feel* any better in the post-meds period, but it did clarify that journeying through these emotions was part of the withdrawal process.

Like Brooke, I had to learn to wade through the intensity of human emotion, which is something I'd never been taught to do—before or after medication. And understanding that those emotions were a normal response to a rough situation made it easier for me to go with the flow, despite how challenging it was.

DEPRESSION AS AN EVOLUTIONARY ADVANTAGE

"THE BASIC IDEA, I think, that I've been working on for roughly twenty years is that depression is probably a normal emotion," says Paul Andrews, an associate professor of evolutionary psychology in the Department of Psychology, Neuroscience, and Behaviour at McMaster University. "With a caveat, which is that the word 'depression' is really a catch-all phrase." Andrews's research interests include ruminative depression—when we think deeply about our distress. There are nine symptoms in the DSM-5 for major depressive disorder (MDD), and one of two that need to be present for a diagnosis include persistent sad or low mood and anhedonia, the inability to find pleasure in things. Individuals can have a combination of the remaining symptoms; for example, some depressed individuals eat and sleep less, while others eat and sleep more.

You don't need to ruminate to meet the DSM-5 symptom criteria for MDD, but rumination is associated with many of the symptoms of depression: guilt, worthlessness, fatigue, and decreased concentration. (When we ruminate, we often lose the ability to concentrate on pleasurable things, like eating or sex.) Andrews sees most cases of ruminative depression as being "normal" in the sense that they are an appropriate response to a situation that requires productive change.

Depression is "an evolutionary paradox," writes Andrews in a 2009 article for *Scientific American*.[21] Why would our brains be prone to malfunction so often if we have evolved to survive and reproduce? To answer this question, Andrews gives me two examples of situations in which individuals might experience symptoms similar to those a depressed person might have. One is when we spike a fever, which is an evolutionary adaptation to defend our bodies against infections. Think about the last time you were sick with a nasty virus. Did you bounce around the house with energy, or did you experience a lack of interest in pleasurable things, low mood, and lethargy or fatigue? You likely rolled yourself into a blanket burrito and did a lot of mindless scrolling on social media.

The other example is starvation, which may initially trigger symptoms of sadness and loss of energy. "When you're a starving organism, the primary problem that you face is finding food," says Andrews. "And you need to migrate often in order to find new food." So, a starving person eventually gets a surge of energy that pushes them toward a resolution of their problem. Andrews proposes that this is an adaptive evolutionary response that ensures the human population continues to proliferate.

Let's now apply this concept of evolutionary adaptation to both depression and anxiety. Our brains and defensive systems have adapted to minimize loss—maybe this is the loss of social support (a fight with a friend or the death of a spouse) or the loss of a job. Our inclination to ruminate on these situations may help to propel us toward a resolution *and* avoid future adversity.[22] If our brains have evolved to respond to social and environmental threats, anxiety can similarly be understood as a helpful response to what our brains predict to be a scary situation.[23]

One example of this is the rising rates of anxiety during the COVID-19 pandemic—a completely appropriate response to an unprecedented and stressful situation. Without anxiety, we might have put ourselves and our family members at risk by not following public health guidelines or not taking appropriate preventative action. Some anxiety is probably a good thing when it comes to protecting our family and wider community.

Andrews tells me a hypothetical story of a surgeon who has made a grave medical error, and a patient has been harmed. To prevent similar errors from occurring again in the future, the clinician must adapt—they will read a patient's chart more carefully, they'll provide better documentation, and perhaps they'll consult a more senior colleague on difficult cases. "Essentially what the research shows is that the more distress they feel, the more likely they make productive changes to their [medical] practice," says Andrews.

A clinician who must overcome a serious medical error through education and skills-based learning is a much different scenario than, for example, a woman who is experiencing intimate partner violence and feels very anxious or depressed—but as in the clinician's case, the distress this woman feels is a logical adaptive response to her situation. As we discussed in previous chapters, this is where social supports and mental health treatments need to come together to provide interventions based on individual and social needs. Instead of treating this woman, and others like her, as though she has a serious mental health condition, doctors instead must be able to ask the right questions, listen, believe their stories, and refer them to women's domestic abuse and violence support services.

Let's assume a scenario where a woman is not experiencing significant trauma or violence but is instead feeling very down in the dumps. We already know that across the board, women are more likely to meet the DSM-5 criteria for depression. Andrews suggests that it could be the ruminative part of the process that plays a bigger role in the difference in diagnosis between women and men. "The sex difference appears to largely be mediated by rumination, which means technically that the reason why [women are] more depressed seems to be that they're ruminating," says Andrews. A 2013 meta-analysis of gender differences in rumination supports this theory. It found that women scored higher on rumination, brooding, and reflection, although it's important to note that the differences between men and women were statistically significant but small.[24]

This aligns with evidence we reviewed in Chapter 3: the female brain may be more susceptible to social threats because of differences in sex hormones and stress response. Fears that we are not being accepted by our peers, or ongoing harassment and bullying, can be turned inward into repetitive patterns of thinking and feeling.

If we turn to findings about our experiences during the pandemic, strong evidence across fifty-nine countries shows that women "tended to be more vulnerable during the pandemic in developing symptoms consistent with various forms of mental disorders such as depression, anxiety and post-traumatic distress."[25] But in response, the authors of this study showed, women were able to use a variety of adaptive coping strategies, which included focusing on doing something about the situation and seeking emotional support from others. In other words, our distress may be higher, but our efforts to make a productive change in response to that distress are also stronger. Essentially, rumination can propel us forward instead of holding us back.

BEAR IN MIND that the idea of women as more emotionally in tune and prone to brooding is likely in part a cultural construct. Kristen Lindquist, who has graced the pages of this book several times, cautions that evolutionary psychology may provide some good insights into depression and anxiety as adaptive responses, but we must be careful that we aren't taking gender stereotypes and trying to justify them through an evolutionary lens.

Understanding that depression and anxiety may be adaptive responses to adversity has been a helpful way for me to reframe my emotions, but even more importantly, I've also learned how my culture has applied its strict and rigid rules to my body. As Lindquist and Feldman write for *Aeon*, I've come to "walk this shoreline where biology and culture meet"[26] to better understand how my experiences have been shaped:

1. *Internally*, as bodily sensations and thoughts; and

2. *Externally*, in the way society applies its norms and rigid standards to my body and my emotions at every stage of my life.

I'm not arguing that by reframing depression and anxiety we can be cured. There is no cure for being human, as the title of Kate Bowler's wise and beautiful book about coming to terms with all of life's joys and pain tells us.[27] The evidence I'm sharing here isn't a treatment for mental illness, but I hope it will broaden our understanding of mental distress. No one ever told me that depression and anxiety can be a *normal response to abnormal situations*. Instead, the message I internalized was that mental illness was my fault, that I would always suffer from it, and that healing wasn't possible.

Making peace with my moods has allowed me to see that my suffering is adaptive, to accept that my response is appropriate, and to then allow myself the time and space to ruminate, as needed. This process has been supported by reframing my emotions and learning to tell myself a different story, which can break the negative self-rumination that I sometimes get stuck in ("I'm no good," "I'll never be able to change," "What's the point," and the many other unhelpful phrases we tell ourselves). Getting off medication is certainly not right for everyone, but for me, it was the catalyst for understanding mental distress beyond a simplistic biological explanation.

None of this happened in a vacuum, and I know that the resources I have gave me the space to examine my emotional distress and find the support I needed. As the wise saying goes, our problems are not our fault, but they are our responsibility—with the caveat that some of us have an easier time taking responsibility for our suffering than others. We do not all have equal choices.

There are days I choose not to be "responsible." I fall back on old coping mechanisms that are objectively not healthy but have served me in the past. On those days, I am gentle with myself, telling myself that I am doing exactly what I need to do to feel safe. But on good days, I have found it easier to reach into my healthy coping toolbox and take out something that serves me well.

11

FROM HYSTERIA
TO HEALING

We do not think ourselves into new ways of living.
We live ourselves into new ways of thinking.

RICHARD ROHR'

FOR MUCH OF THIS BOOK, I have focused on structural and
social issues related to our emotional well-being, and I have
hopefully driven home the point that our mental health
crisis cannot be solved by placing all the responsibility on
the individual. Much of mental illness has essentially been
caused by patriarchy, capitalism, and white supremacy, and
clearly seeing how inequality makes us sick is a vital step
toward tackling the extent of the problem. As Emily and
Amelia Nagoski write in their book *Burnout: The Secret to
Unlocking the Stress Cycle*, "Looking at the scale and scope of
the rigging can be painful—scary and enraging and overwhelming. No wonder people hate the word 'patriarchy.'
It's a word that exposes and names a source of pain so old
and deep we've learned to ignore it or treat it as if it's how

life should be."[2] This book may have felt overwhelming to read at times, because there are no easy answers or ten-step solutions.

That being said, as I proposed earlier, there are individual methods that can improve well-being and be helpful supports when we feel overwhelmed. In this final chapter, I share some of the paths that women can take toward embodiment—a process that helps us to recognize ourselves as whole human beings worthy of care. In her book *The Wisdom of Your Body: Finding Healing, Wholeness, and Connection Through Embodied Living*, author Hillary McBride defines embodiment as "the experience of being a body in a social context."[3] Learning embodiment has changed me and helped me to heal, but I have also had to learn the ways in which my culture would prefer I stay disembodied and the ways I am taught to ignore my intuition and close myself off to the connection I have with other bodies.

These strategies are much more about shedding the things you may have learned than about amassing more knowledge or self-care strategies. This is about a greater reliance on yourself as someone who already knows what needs to be done. It isn't intended to be prescriptive, and I recognize that we are all living with different capacities and differing abilities to face adversity. Some of these things may be accessible to you, and they may fit well in your life, while others may seem pointless, difficult, or impossible. While I believe that embodiment is the crucial piece of the puzzle that many women are missing, both individually and socially, there are many ways to get there.

This is also where I get to highlight research into aspects of human well-being that we are only just beginning to study and understand. On the molecular level, I explore the connection between our microbes and our brains and how this bidirectional relationship may hold the key to better mental health. I then meander out to the limbs of the body and mind, through the practices of yoga and meditation. Beyond the body is the space we inhabit, the wilderness outside our front doors, which may bring us more peace than we ever imagined. Finally, I explore the ineffable joy to be found in spirituality and creativity, in our search for the sacredness and purpose of life. Much of this research is in its infancy, and while some results are promising, it is too early to declare things like body movement, time in the outdoors, and probiotics as cure-alls for psychiatric illnesses. (And I don't think they ever will be, since mental illness is multi-faceted and calls for a multifaceted treatment approach.) For now, we can learn to rely on what feels good and true to ourselves and our personal capacity for creating change.

GUT SENSE: THE MICROBIOME AND OUR MOODS

IN THE EARLY YEARS of my mental health crisis, I was always willing to try the new big thing on the market that claimed to lessen anxiety and depression. Alternative medicine is a massive industry in the West, a testament to how far we will go when we feel that the established medical system has failed us, or when we have exhausted all the options that modern medicine can offer. That said, there are valid concerns from mainstream medical practitioners that patients are putting themselves at risk by trying treatments that have not been well studied.

In my teens, I wasn't worried about good scientific evidence, so I was a regular customer of the supplement aisle at the local health food store near my home. I tried St. John's wort, valerian, and many other supplements that probably drained my parents' bank account but didn't have any noticeable effect on my anxiety.

One day I carted home a box of drinkable dairy probiotics, which I choked down every morning before breakfast. I had little hope for this pasty white goo, which tasted like sour milk and resembled baby spit-up. But over several weeks, while my anxiety didn't improve much, I did notice a significant difference in my gastrointestinal issues. I'd contracted several viruses in the previous school year, but I didn't get sick once in the months that I diligently took my morning probiotics.

It was a nineteenth-century microbiologist and Nobel laureate, Élie Metchnikoff, who noticed that people who consumed fermented milk products appeared to be healthier and lived longer.[4] Our guts contain an estimated one thousand different species of bacteria, and some of these were being commercially manufactured by companies as early as the 1920s.[5] Despite claims that ingesting these bacteria would support health and vitality, prior to the 2000s, very little research had been done to explore the link between supplemental bacteria and our moods.

A review of thirty-four studies (on both prebiotics and probiotics) found a small but significant difference in the mental health of participants taking probiotics for depression and anxiety. However, many of the trials excluded people who had clinically diagnosed anxiety and depression, featuring a general population from the community instead.[6] The small number of trials that did study psychiatric populations showed greater effects for the probiotics when compared to a placebo, and the authors concluded that more studies are needed for these specific populations.

To explore the connection between our gut and our mental health, I reached out to Kara Gross Margolis, an associate professor and director for gut-brain science at the New York University Pain Research Center, and an expert in gut-brain axis disorders. Margolis has studied how neurotransmitters, like serotonin and oxytocin, play a role in our enteric nervous system ("enteric" means relating to or affecting the intestines). "The brain-gut axis is a relationship between the brain and the gut," she says. "It's a communication that happens twenty-four hours a day, seven days a week, and is bidirectional." In other words, the brain sends signals to the gut, and the gut also influences the way the brain operates and behaves.

Margolis says that the main highway of communication between these two partners is the vagus nerve, and it appears that about three-quarters of all this communication is traveling from the gut to the brain. "The gut serves as a sensory organ or as an entry point for recognizing different things that are happening in our environment, at least at the level of the gut," she says.

Because of this two-way communication, it's been difficult for experts to determine the source of problems affecting the brain or the gut. Do people with gastrointestinal (GI) problems go on to develop mood disorders, or do people who first have mood disorders develop GI problems? It's a question I'm very interested in answering, because my mental illness was always tangled up with abdominal distress.

Margolis says that studies show the majority of patients who started with GI disorders (but no anxiety and depression) end up developing anxiety and depression, while some patients who have psychiatric conditions do go on to develop GI disorders. "It's a real conundrum," she says.

This link between the gut and the brain is likely to become an even greater focus of future therapies. Neurotransmitters like serotonin, produced mainly in the gut under the influence of our gut microbiota (all the microorganisms found there), can make pit stops along the vagus nerve to activate receptors that engage the parasympathetic nervous system in the process of "rest and digest." This helps to lower our heart rate, slow respiration, and improve digestion—like a built-in chill pill for the body.[7]

Commercial interests have already made a play at cashing in on this novel understanding of our gut-brain connection. "There's a lot of stuff on the web about increasing serotonin in your diet or taking serotonin supplements over the counter," Margolis says. The problem with taking oral supplements, she says, is that our body has very tight controls in place: when cells release serotonin, our system quickly moves to inactivate it so that the receptors don't become overstimulated. This is important, because serotonin has many effects on the gut, the brain, the lungs, the kidneys, and the immune system. "So, if you take something that gives a standard serotonin dose or you eat a meal high in tryptophan, which is the building block of serotonin—like turkey—serotonin will be created in the gut. But it will be sucked up and inactivated too quickly to work in some of the ways it is commercialized to help— for example, mood."

Margolis doesn't begrudge anyone's willingness to try a supplement, even if it only results in a placebo effect. "But from the studies we have to date, there's nothing that would show that the supplement works," she says.

In her research, Margolis has formulated and then studied the effects of a form of serotonin that releases slowly and continuously in the gut, using up the ability of the transporter to suck it back up, meaning that some of it remains in the gut and the brain longer.[8] This formulation has been tested in mice, but there is work by another group of researchers to move to phase one trials in humans.

Although there's still so much we don't know about the brain-gut axis, Margolis says there have been tremendous advances in the field. "I think someday we're going to be able to poop into a cup and our microbiome and metabolome are going to be analyzed ... and we're going to be able to tailor specially made bacteria that can produce specific neurotransmitters that can help the gut and the brain," she says. She sees bioengineered microbiota as a key treatment in the future of personalized medicine.

Early stages of this idea are already underway, and commercial interest in microbiome testing is growing. Companies ask you to fill out some forms, poop in a cup, and mail in your sample—for a cost, of course. In return, you receive a report, which analyzes your gut bacteria in relation to various diseases and disorders.[9] One website I looked up told me that a "full body intelligence test" of my microbiome would help me "unlock [my] body's innate ability to restore health and boost longevity at a molecular level."[10] With this field of study still in its early stages, I don't think I'll be forking out my hard-earned cash anytime soon.

As for supplemental probiotics, whether or not choking down gooey yogurt each day boosts my mood remains unclear. Studies have shown some promising but limited findings, with evidence that may not be applicable to diverse populations, the many different bacterial strains available, and different dosages and durations of treatment.[11] As with almost all topics covered in this chapter, more and better-quality research is needed—and it will be exciting to see where it takes us.

FEELING BLUE? HAVE YOU TRIED YOGA AND MEDITATION?

IF YOU'VE NEVER RECEIVED advice to just do yoga and meditate for your mental health, congratulations, because you are probably one of only a handful of people who have avoided this suggestion (and maybe you live under a rock?). I was told time and again to "do yoga and breathe deeply," and in my younger years, I found the advice to be annoying and simplistic. If yoga and meditation worked, wouldn't I have seen *some* improvement in my symptoms? Little did I know that these practices take years to master, and many people do indeed experience a mental health boost over time. The key may be finding the right kind of practice, because they're not all equally effective for every individual.

I started my first yoga class at a local community center, during the time of my teenage breakdown. I can't remember the teacher's credentials or what flavor of yoga she was teaching, but I know it mostly focused on a single "limb" of yoga called "asana." This is the physical practice that most people encounter in a typical yoga class in the West, and it includes poses like the downward dog and cat-cow. As I would later discover, the other limbs of yoga are meant to guide the participant down a path to freedom and enlightenment and involve much more than shaping your body into an ideal posture. The roots of the practice extend well beyond the mat to encompass morals and values and wide-ranging practices of health and education.

Yoga and meditation are cultural and religious practices, but in the West, they have also come to serve a growing number of people seeking both fitness and a way to cope with the stress of modern life. In my twenties, I took my first mindfulness-based stress reduction (MBSR) program, a course created by Jon Kabat-Zinn, who adapted Buddhist mindfulness teachings for North Americans. Kabat-Zinn has received criticism for Westernizing traditional Eastern practices, but he has always maintained that his program is "anchored in the ethical framework that lies at the very heart of the original teachings of the Buddha." It also, he contends, provides an important opportunity to address the many sources of pain and suffering in our modern world.[12]

My course was led by a psychotherapist and mindfulness teacher, who collected before-and-after measures of depression and anxiety symptoms. MBSR involves a weekly two-and-a-half-hour group class, daily meditation and yoga practices, and a full-day weekend retreat. I stuck to the program religiously, and after eight weeks, the results that my teacher shared with me were indeed significant—where I had previously rated my mood and functioning as poor, many of those scores had shifted to the more positive end of the scale after completing the program. (Participants' results have not been published, as they were meant to be shared only with participants and their physicians; however, my teacher, Bill Knight, did share a cost-effectiveness study with me, which showed that MBSR participants had lower health care utilization one year after the program was completed.) [13]

Almost twenty years later, I still feel the positive impact that this course has had on my mental health. MBSR laid a solid foundation for the rebuilding I needed to do, and it was the first time I practiced embodiment—learning how to just be in my body and work with moment-by-moment awareness of my bodily sensations and my thoughts. I consider it my starting point when I look back on my journey of healing.

In my work as a freelance writer, I became interested in the science of mindfulness, which has seen exponential growth since the earliest Western publication in the mid-1960s. [14] The body of literature suggests that mindfulness can be beneficial for a range of physical and mental health outcomes, though the majority of this scientific work comes from the West. [15] In a recent trial comparing a common antidepressant (escitalopram, or Lexapro) to MBSR, the researchers found that mindfulness was just as effective as the drug in reducing anxiety, and came with fewer side effects. [16]

The science of yoga has experienced a similar proliferation. Heather Mason, founder of the Minded Institute, a yoga therapy training program for professionals who work with people with mental and physical health conditions, tells me about a study that suggests that yoga can increase GABA levels in the brain and improve mood and anxiety. (GABA is a neurotransmitter that can lessen a nerve cell's ability to receive or transmit signals to another cell.) Compared to a randomly assigned group who went for a walk three times a week, the people practicing yoga postures over twelve weeks reported greater improvement in mood and a decrease in anxiety. There was also a stronger relationship between the yoga group's mental health benefits and GABA levels (measured using an imaging technique on one part of the brain), which means they found a correlation between better mood and increased levels of GABA.[17]

Mason says that GABA helps to inhibit neural pathways associated with fear, and people with anxiety have low GABA levels (which could be why we have a more fearful response to stressful situations). Other research has assessed possible biomarkers that could predict clinical improvement in people with psychiatric disorders who participate in yoga, and results are promising.[18]

An older meta-analysis from 2011 included ten studies on yoga therapy; the result was significant for yoga-based interventions (compared to a control group) in the treatment of major psychiatric disorders. However, the review did not assess the quality of the trials, and some of the studies included participants who had not been diagnosed with mental illness.[19] The control groups were not well reported, so it's hard to tease out what yoga was being compared to. A more recent review that did assess study quality found that yoga may be beneficial as a stand-alone or complementary therapy in the treatment of depression, but the effectiveness of yoga for PTSD was unclear.[20] Taken together, we can say that these are promising results, but the field could really benefit from well-designed and higher-quality trials, which would help convince the medical community to embrace yoga's potential.

There are hundreds of different yoga and meditation programs, workshops, or apps available to people who live in Western countries, and finding the best fit can take some trial and error. One of the critiques of Westernized forms of yoga and mindfulness is that they are too elitist, pushing away groups for whom these practices are part of their religious traditions. In an article for *Vice*, Kendra Surmitis, a professor of counseling at Prescott College, says that she tries to educate people on the roots of the mindfulness practices they're exploring. "I would encourage practitioners to request the mentorship or support of someone who is most familiar with the background of the practice, such as a Buddhist monastic," she says, "to assist them in truly understanding the history of the practice, its spiritual relevance, and how this ought to be communicated to the larger population."[21]

For those who are new to mindfulness and meditation, seeking out a trained teacher who can answer questions and guide you through any difficulties can be supportive. Most cities in North America have meditation centers that provide classes on a donation basis or offer bursaries for courses like MBSR, which expands the accessibility of these programs.

For women especially, how we pay attention to our physical selves and move our bodies—the specific setting and practice—has a profound impact on how we integrate that knowledge as we seek emotional well-being. Given the high rates of trauma and sexual abuse that women have experienced, it may be a good idea to scope out yoga and meditation courses where the teacher has specific trauma-related training.

I WENT ON to take other courses in meditation and yoga, some of which were based in cultural traditions and others that were very much Westernized versions. At times, I struggled with being told exactly *how* to practice mindfulness, through long periods of sitting on a cushion, keeping my eyes closed, and becoming peacefully aware of my body and surroundings. Likewise, some yoga classes felt more like intense exercise and led to pain and injury rather than the peace and balance I was seeking.

During an appointment with my therapist, I discussed the conflicted relationship I had with yoga, and I used my experience with the happy baby pose as an example. This yoga pose asks you to lie on your back and grab hold of your toes, just like a baby on the changing table. The pose used to make me angry and tearful, and I had no idea why. My reaction was maybe related to my inflexibility thwarting my desire to force myself into the same posture as everyone else in class; or maybe it was something else that I had yet to learn or acknowledge about myself. Either way, it was not a posture that I enjoyed, and I ended up feeling vulnerable and afraid.

After I described all this, my therapist asked me why I couldn't just do a different pose or get up off the mat and go for a walk. I stopped to think for a moment and asked myself why I felt compelled to stay in a position that clearly wasn't working. My therapist helped me to realize that I am in control; no one can force me into an uncomfortable position, and I didn't have to subject myself to something that didn't feel safe.

Yoga and mindfulness continue to play an important role in my own well-being, but I no longer follow a class blindly without regard for my emotional and physical safety. If a movement feels wrong or hurts, I stop. This is easy to do at home, but in a public class, I still get that strong urge to follow the crowd. I'm learning to acknowledge my bodily autonomy and work through those feelings of wanting to please the teacher or keep up with the class. More often than not, I am able to stop myself and lie quietly on my mat while the rest of the class finishes their posture.

I have branched out from these practices to find other forms of body movement, some of which don't subscribe to any one tradition or culture. Dance classes like Zumba have been enormously fun and healing for me, and I enjoy doing them in settings that are inclusive of all body types, all genders, and all levels of coordination. I practice mindfulness now throughout my day, tapping into my breathing and bodily sensations while I complete mundane tasks like washing the dishes or folding laundry. I still do the occasional meditation "on a cushion" when I think my body could benefit from some dedicated quiet time, but I've learned to listen to my own intuition on what feels right in the moment. Giving myself the freedom to choose parts of different traditions and piece together my own style of practice has been a better way for me to learn to trust my body and understand what it needs at different moments of my life.

NATURE AS HEALER

THE WIND IS LIGHT TODAY, taking a lazy brush over the teal surface of the lake. I step one foot into the water, then the other foot, bracing myself for impact. I put my arms over my head and dive, surfacing beyond the buoy line of the sandy beach. The waves are bigger the deeper I go, and occasionally I get a smack in the face and a mouthful of refreshing lake tang.

Soon I'm in the center of the lake, alone with the water striders, which scoot away from me on their long and spindly legs as my hands cut through the surface of the water. My breathing settles and my thoughts fall away as I focus on the movement of my legs and arms, propelling me forward. The sun strains to break through the marshmallow clouds, its weak rays reflecting off the surface of the water.

If there is anything as peaceful as this, I have yet to discover it.

Melissa Lem, a Vancouver family physician and longtime advocate of the health benefits of nature, remembers feeling that same quieting effect while spending time in the outdoors. (Lem and I went to high school together, and I'm delighted that she agreed to speak with me for this book.) "I grew up feeling that connection to nature and not necessarily feeling as connected to my community as I should have been," she tells me. She experienced racism and bullying on the playground and at school. "I found when I spent time at the park or when our family would go camping in Bruce Peninsula National Park... I felt so comfortable. I didn't feel like anyone was going to come and yell something at me or exclude me."

Lem tells me about facing other stressors in her early career as a doctor, and the way nature improved her mental health. In her first role, as a rural family physician in Northern British Columbia, she faced intensive work running an emergency room and performing acute care during long overnight shifts. Despite the challenges, she loved the work and credits easy access to nature as part of what helped her cope. "My commute was walking to work past the hospital garden and looking at the mist rising over the mountains—I think that went a long way," she says.

Then she moved to the busy metropolis of Toronto, which she describes as "streetcar town, skyscrapers, and concrete."

Suddenly she found herself much more stressed, even though her work was easier than in B.C. After she realized that her problem was a lack of access to the great outdoors, she decided to do a literature review to collect evidence that would support her intuitive sense that nature was a missing piece of the well-being puzzle. "It had to be backed up by evidence, because I'm a doctor trained in evidence-based medicine," she says. What Lem found was a large body of literature on the health benefits of nature, which she says none of her colleagues were talking about at the time.

A systematic review from 2018 included 143 studies on the topic from the previous decade, illustrating a recent and rapid growth in the study of nature and health.[22] A quick search on PubMed for citations since 2018 gave me over two thousand results for "greenspace and health," with that number growing year over year.

It's not just the wilds of the forest that have been studied. The systematic review I reference above included studies of eleven different types of greenspace, such as urban trees and street greenery, larger parks, forests, and even the effect of viewing trees from a hospital room window. The review found statistically significant benefits for a heap of objective (and some self-reported) health measures, including all-cause mortality, type 2 diabetes, measures of cardiovascular health, blood pressure, stress hormone levels, and preterm birth.

There are also many studies showing that nature can be therapeutic for those with mental health challenges, including reviews on horticulture therapy[23] and wilderness adventure therapy for young people.[24] What we don't yet fully understand are the underlying reasons *why* greenspace might benefit our mental well-being, which means we don't know enough about how to replicate these interventions for different populations. Would gardening be something teens would want to do? Could wilderness adventure therapy work for older people with physical limitations?

"A doctor prescribing nature time in Regent Park is different from a doctor prescribing nature in Kitsilano, so we have to definitely be aware of our patients' strengths and abilities, and also the communities we live in," says Lem, comparing a low-income housing community in Toronto with a trendy neighborhood in Vancouver surrounded by beautiful biodiversity. Lack of access to nature is a problem, with many people living in urban gray areas where scraggly trees barely survive in a concrete desert. "We're coming up with a plan for programs where people can get free or discounted transit to greenspaces to reduce that barrier," she says, adding that it's also important to change people's perceptions of what nature can be. "You don't have to be in the middle of a forest by yourself or on the side of a mountain; it can be in your garden or your neighborhood park."

IT WAS A NATUROPATHIC DOCTOR (ND) who handed me my first PaRx—a park prescription, sometimes called a ParkRx or NatureRx. I had exhausted all the treatment options with my family doctor and had turned to alternative medicine for answers. In addition to several nutritional supplements and dietary changes, my ND suggested I leave my claustrophobic cubicle each day at lunchtime, head over to a small butterfly garden adjacent to our office building, and take off my shoes. I was to stand in the grass for ten minutes, feeling the cool blades tickling my toes. This was written down on an actual prescription pad, and I carried the slip home with me in my bag.

The prescription felt silly at first, but I dutifully followed it every day throughout that summer. I would burst out of the air-conditioned building at lunchtime into a wave of oppressive heat, my eyes adjusting from fake fluorescent lighting to the stunning white glare of the sun. I'd shuffle around in the grass while other employees lounged near the garden eating their lunch. And I was surprised to find that it helped—my lunchtime communion with this small greenspace seemed to set the tone for a better mood in the afternoon and post-work evening. I began to look for other ways to incorporate the outdoors into my everyday life, like biking to work instead of taking the bus. I went for daily walks in the ravine behind my house.

Nature prescriptions, or "nature pills," are a growing area of interest for researchers and medical practitioners. Lem is one of the leaders in the movement in Canada and has launched the Park Prescriptions (PaRx) initiative with the BC Parks Foundation, a program offering health care professionals nature prescription files and codes, with instructions for how to write and log their nature prescriptions. "There are just under 100,000 physicians in Canada, and over 5000 registered for our program, so that's over 5 percent of doctors," she says. "I think it's important for nature to become routine advice during a health care visit—diet, exercise, sleep, and nature time." Lem calls these the four central pillars of health, and she's excited to see the movement growing among physicians.

PaRx is not just a movement; it's also a treatment practice backed by science. In one study of thirty-six urban residents

(92 percent of whom identified as women), participants were prescribed a nature pill over eight weeks; they were instructed to engage in a nature experience three days per week, for a minimum duration of ten minutes. The experience could be anywhere outside where there were enough natural elements for the participant to feel like they were interacting with nature. The researchers collected before-and-after saliva samples and found that time in nature produced a 21.3 percent per hour decrease in cortisol levels, with the best outcomes from nature pills with a duration of twenty to thirty minutes.[25]

It is important to note that this was a small study and participants self-selected, meaning they were open and willing to spend time in nature, which doesn't help to answer the question of whether less-willing people would experience similar benefits. But it is convincing nonetheless, and the study joins a growing body of knowledge that tells us the PaRx movement might be on to something.

I CONNECT MY OWN TIME in nature to similar benefits I get from practicing mindfulness. I believe that it's not just about the trees that I'm seeing or the cold water that's lapping around me. The setting becomes the doorway to a deeper connection with my body, which gives me the space I need to mindfully observe all the things happening within and around me—something I wouldn't be able to tap into if I were distracted by my phone or hurrying through a park to get to a destination. The science agrees with me: the mindful component of time in the outdoors could be one of the key reasons we experience such significant changes in our psychological and physiological health.[26]

Other research suggests that it's not only the positive health outcome that we get from nature that is the interesting part—it's what *predicts* those positive changes. In the example of my cold lake swim, being in the presence of something awe-inspiring could be what's causing real physical changes in my body.

DOING SPIRITUALITY YOUR WAY

LIKE YOGA, MINDFULNESS, and the great outdoors, the role of spirituality as a contributor to good mental health has largely remained on the periphery of scientific inquiry. Anecdotally, some of us may know or suspect that our spirituality can make us feel better or worse, depending on the context of our beliefs and the experiences we've had in religious groups. While the connection between spirituality and well-being has been studied in many different parts of the world (and publications on these topics have rapidly expanded), Western psychiatry has not done as thorough a job embracing the potential of spirituality.[27]

David Rosmarin, a psychiatric researcher who has studied spirituality and mental health, writes that spirituality "encompasses connection—religious or otherwise—with a non-physical reality as perceived by the individual."[28] It's a connection that's felt by billions of people around the world, and yet a story we often hear in the media is that religious affiliation is on the decline. Indeed, research does underscore a downward shift in the numbers of individuals who identify with a specific religion in North America[29] and who identify as "practicing" in western Europe.[30] In other countries and regions, religious belief is ticking upward, with Islam being the fastest growing religion in the world.[31]

Many individuals in North America identify themselves as unaffiliated with a specific religion but still believe in God or a personally defined higher power. And this demographic is rapidly growing in the United States, making up 27 percent of the population in 2017.[32] Researchers have called for funding and future study to focus on this burgeoning group, to better understand the mental health needs of these individuals and to begin collecting international data to track how religious or spiritual identities vary from country to country.[33] One study found that people who report being spiritual, but not religious, may be more vulnerable to mental disorders.[34] However, the data on mental health and religiosity is almost always self-reported and collected at one time in a person's life, which means no firm conclusions can be made about causality.

What we can surmise from the literature is that components of religion and spirituality may give humans a sense of structure and meaning, which is certainly more comforting than chaos or lack of meaning. Religion also offers hope during challenging times, and most traditions have practices of compassion and forgiveness that can be directed toward the self or to others. Religious individuals seem to better cope with stress and have lower rates of depression, suicide, anxiety, and substance use.[35] One review on the effects of religiosity and spirituality on mental health among cancer patients also found a positive association, although the authors call for more research on what it is about these practices that leads to better mental health.[36] Is it the sense of community? The practice of prayer, which can be very meditative? Specific moral teachings that may discourage behaviors like drinking or recreational drug-taking?

Some of the benefits could have a lot to do with the link between our spiritual and religious identity and our brain. An exciting body of research in the field of neurotheology is on the specific mechanisms of action (*why* and *how* spirituality affects our mental health) and seeks to explore the ways that certain practices, like chanting or prayer, affect brain networks and neurotransmitter systems.[37] One study on the effect of a spiritual retreat showed significant brain changes in participants' functional connectivity in the areas of the brain that release serotonin and dopamine.[38]

While spirituality-based interventions to support mental health are few and far between, those that I found are adapted from CBT-based methods. These methods involve concrete direction from the therapist for the patient to explore their spiritual or religious beliefs through activities like prayer or reading religious texts, performing good deeds, or counting blessings (a bit like a secular gratitude practice). Studies on these methods do show promising results,[39] and recent work has highlighted the fact that many patients desire a spiritual component in therapy.[40]

Providing spiritual-based therapy does come with some risks for people who have a history of religious trauma. It's imperative for therapists to better understand the emotional push-pull of spiritual and religious life, especially as it relates to girls, women, and gender-diverse people, who have historically experienced more harm from religious cultures. In her master's thesis on religious trauma, Jolyn Sloan, a counselor living in British Columbia, writes, "Many mental health practitioners may feel uncomfortable incorporating religious or spiritual beliefs in their practice because of their own disconnection to spiritual issues. I argue that mental health practitioners do not need to be experts in the theology of their clients. They are invited to understand the intense cognitive and emotional distress one can experience when transitioning out of their fundamentalist beliefs and community and be willing to have genuine, caring conversations about spiritual and religious issues. Mental health practitioners also need to be able to help those people affected reconstruct another worldview."[41]

I GREW UP IN A SOCIAL CIRCLE that was skeptical of religion. It was okay to drive around with a shiny cross dangling from your rearview mirror, but that's as far as the tolerance went for religious belief. Attending church or temple, reading religious texts, or talking about the divine was *not* something people welcomed with open arms. Only in my adult years have I been able to accept that spirituality is vital to my well-being. When I say that spirituality has improved my mental health, I don't mean that connecting to some higher power has cured me of my human predisposition to anxiety and depression. Instead, it's helped me tap into two important aspects of my emotional life: awe and expansiveness.

Awe is an under-studied and, some might say, undervalued emotion. As Deborah Farmer Kris writes in the *Washington Post*, "Awe is what we feel when we encounter something vast, wondrous or beyond our ordinary frame of reference. It evokes a sense of mystery and wonder."[42] In a study of positive emotions and blood markers of inflammation in the body, the researchers discovered that the emotion of awe (among six other positive emotions)

was the strongest predictor of lower levels of inflammatory markers.[43] Of course, we're not sure if awe decreases
inflammation or whether people with less inflammation are
more likely to experience awe, but it's an exciting avenue of
future research.

Experiencing awe specifically in nature may also have
healing benefits, which is why I think some people call
nature their religion. In his book *Chatter: The Voice in Our
Head, Why It Matters, and How to Harness It*, Ethan Kross
documents the experience of veteran Suzanne Bott. She
participated in a study led by a research team at the University of California, Berkeley, which sent military veterans
and youth from underserved communities on a four-day
whitewater rafting trip. The results showed that Bott and her
travel companions experienced reductions in their stress and
PTSD levels and felt happier and more satisfied.[44] What pre-
dicted these changes above and beyond all the other positive
emotions studied was a sense of awe. Kross writes, "When
you're in the presence of something vast and indescribable
it's hard to maintain the view that you—and the voice in
your head—are the center of the world ... When you feel
smaller in the midst of awe-inspiring sights—a phenomenon
described as a 'shrinking of the self'—so do your problems."[45]

I remember numerous experiences of awe as a child.
Many of these occurred in nature when the sacredness of
our earthly lives would hit me with a sudden jolt: blood-red
sunsets, harvest moons, freshly fallen snow on tree boughs,
the reflection of sky on water, or the chill of a sky full of stars.
A sense of awe has also come over me in my adult life: in
my work as a birth doula, welcoming tiny newborn miracles
into the world, or in quiet moments of meditation, when

the perspective on my body shifts and suddenly I am a tiny speck drifting through the infinite universe.

This shifting perspective illuminates the expansiveness of life, that my connection with other humans and with the earth is rich and vast. A sense of awe and expansiveness can be discovered through our five senses, bringing us into our bodies, as well as into a connection with other bodies and other living things. If you've ever felt the rush of goosebumps up your arms while listening to a beautiful song, you've felt awe. Whether you call this "God" or "magic" or "emotion" doesn't matter all that much. What matters is how it helps us to live our lives by igniting a sense of wonder, which I think allows us to be gentler to ourselves and one another, and to honor the mystery in our lives.

There may be one final practice that has similar benefits for the body, and it's similarly linked to the shrinking of the self—but in a way that brings us closer to a state of deep concentration and wild creativity.

GETTING CURIOUS
ABOUT CREATIVITY

IN THERAPY WE ARE OFTEN ASKED to think of a place or time when we've felt truly at peace, so that we can go to that place in times of stress. During a panic attack, we might close our eyes and conjure up a windswept beach and the rhythmic sound of crashing waves. It's an exercise that helps to soothe the nervous system and bring us back to simpler times, when we didn't feel the chaotic push and pull of our emotions.

When I've been asked to name a happy place from my childhood, I think of creative times: raising my instrument to create a gorgeous symphony of sound in my youth orchestra, or the peacefulness of Saturday morning art classes—getting lost in a chunk of uninterrupted time, hands caked in dried clay or smeared in blue paint. When I was left with time to myself, I was drawn into the current of flow, a concept first introduced by psychologist Mihaly Csikszentmihalyi to describe the experience "during which individuals are fully involved in the present moment."[46]

In her book *Find Your Unicorn Space: Reclaim Your Creative Life in a Too-Busy World*, author Eve Rodsky describes flow as being made up of two important factors: uninterrupted time and sustained attention to an activity you love.[47] In a state of flow, our attention is so absorbed by the task at hand that time becomes distorted, and before we know it, we've forgotten to stop for lunch.

Another component of flow that I find even more fascinating is what researchers Jeanne Nakamura and Csikszentmihalyi note as the loss of self-consciousness, or the awareness of ourselves as the ones doing the creating. I think this ties in nicely with the theory of the diminished self in the emotional experience of awe.[48] Becoming *un*conscious of these different components of our self allows us moments of freedom from those pesky dictators on our shoulders who tell us who to be and how to act—our genes and our culture. The intense concentration that's required for a creative activity allows us to let go of the "me, me, me" thinking we regularly engage in, as our attention is taken up entirely by the task at hand.

"But wait," you might be saying. "Didn't you say earlier that embodiment and knowledge of our internal state is a key piece of building better emotional health?" I absolutely did, and I think especially for girls and women who have learned to ignore or dismiss their body's messages, a good starting place is how we feel in our bodies.

But as you unlock that level of knowledge, there are benefits to regularly shifting the focus of your attention to something external. If your consciousness is an awareness of all those different selves—the internal body experience, memories, genes, and culture—then where you choose to place your limited attention can change the experience of your *whole* self. In their writing on flow, Nakamura and Csikszentmihalyi quote psychologist William James as saying, "*My experience is what I agree to attend to.* Only those items which I *notice* shape my mind" (and, I would add, shape our bodies as well).[49]

By focusing attention on a creative pursuit, women may learn to let go of expectations and discover a true sense of freedom. Creativity is the ultimate expression of self in a world that demands our conformity.

JOANNE LAUZON, AN ARTIST and creative play coach living in Ottawa, says that it took her many years before she realized she was using creativity as a form of self-care. Lauzon grew up in a home with a lot of conflict, and she remembers taking refuge in her room and doodling on a notepad. "Looking back, I realized that was a form of escape for me, just to get out of the situation in the house and tap into the flow state as a form of healing."

As an adult, much of her career was focused on graphic design, but she always had a sketchpad or two on the go and did some form of creative play as a way to get "out of her head" for a few moments. When she started sharing her work on Instagram, people (mostly women) responded by asking her to teach them unique skills of hand-lettering, calligraphy, and watercolor painting. "Now I can't stand it when someone calls me an art teacher," she says, "because I want to promote the benefits of creativity as a form of self-care and healing."

It was in those first few workshops that it became obvious to Lauzon that many women really struggle to let go and fall into that flow state. "They needed whatever it was they were doing to be right, to be perfect, or to be good enough—and of course, those are all words that we use to describe ourselves," she says. Lauzon began having conversations with women as they sat around her studio table, asking them to explore their rigid thinking about the art they were creating. "Learning how to tap into their creative energy and use it as a way to connect to themselves and connect to their bodies gave their nervous system a chance to relax," she says.

When we're actively choosing to give our attention to creative flow, research has also shown that this results in positive affect, another term for those good vibes that can counteract stress and anxiety.[50] And this is where Lauzon has seen significant healing take place. She remembers one woman who attended her five-week course who was grieving the loss of her partner and also dealing with significant health issues. "She came to me in the second week and said, 'I just wanted to say to you that I have no joy in my life, and I'm really hoping that you can help me find that through these classes.'" She's since done multiple retreats and courses with Lauzon, and she now laughs all the time, wears brighter colors, and is doing more adventurous things. "She often says thank you to me for holding her hand through those scary moments of growth and self-discovery and for letting her play in an environment with no judgment," says Lauzon.

Indeed, creativity and the act of play go hand in hand. Eve Rodsky points out that creativity has a lot to do with curiosity, and that it's "not just limited to the 'making' (of visual art or creative writing). It is also 'developing' (a new skill set), 'expanding' (your knowledge within your area of expertise), and 'learning' (of advancements in your fields of interest) and more. Meaning, you don't have to pick up a paintbrush to express your creativity!"[51]

Regardless of the type of creative pursuit you are drawn to, not all moments of creativity give rise to a creative flow state. It's possible to be creative at work or in our home lives, but that's not necessarily going to help us feel less bored, anxious, or depressed. For example, I've had to be creative all the time with my kids, coming up with novel solutions to parenting challenges, like how to get my toddler to put on socks or my middle-schooler to wear her coat. In my past role as a researcher, I engaged in creativity when I sat down with large reams of data and came up with ways to analyze that data and write an engaging report or journal article on my findings. In neither of those situations have I felt particularly happy or rewarded by my abilities.

Of course, our ability to reach flow state relies on our personal time capacity and, more specifically, time when we won't be interrupted by the needs of others. As we covered in Chapter 7, most women watch the opportunity for uninterrupted time slip through their fingertips as they attend to jobs, kids, and housework.

Scientific studies have observed inequalities with respect to the amount of time that men and women spend on leisure.

A study on 869 young adults found that in a single day, women dedicate less time to leisure activities compared with men.[52] An American time-use survey found that fathers spend about three hours more in leisure time than mothers per week (27.5 versus 24.5 hours), and this pattern is similar in countries around the world.[53] But in these two studies, the data showed that although women had less time for leisure overall, they seemed to derive more satisfaction from it.

"We're already overwhelmed with so many other baskets in our daily life, and adding creativity to that is just one more thing" says Lauzon. "That's an objection that I come up against a lot." To address this, Lauzon says that she follows American entrepreneur Marie Forleo's advice "to create before you consume": when you wake up in the morning, do something creative before consuming information from the outside world. Like self-care, creativity doesn't have to be consumerist: we can be creative at home without buying any products.

Lauzon also says that making time for creativity puts us into that flow state, which can make us better able to withstand the onslaught from our daily lives. "Having time of healing and connection to the self makes you more resilient, and more of a problem-solver," she says. "If I can hit people over the head with one message, it would be that we all have creative energy—we make creative choices every single day."

For women, this is a time to reclaim our creativity—as a birthright and not a skill to be gained. Creativity is in the essence and the truest expression of yourself.

I REALIZE I'VE ONLY skimmed the surface of individual-level strategies that can carry us through difficult days. There isn't yet enough evidence from a Western science perspective to justify funding these alternatives on a large scale, but my hope is that smaller-scale and community-based options can fill the gap—at least until our understanding of mind-body therapeutics advances.

It's worth noting that many of us tell stories about our individual recovery from mental illness in ways that point to our continuing preoccupation with managing our mental health through coping strategies, mindset, and fierce resolve. As a culture, we are drawn to the shiniest stories: the ones in which the person has achieved success in the bare capitalist sense—they are well enough to hold down a job, raise a family, and contribute to society. This makes the stories of those who can't work or choose not to have children due to their mental illness invisible.

We all love a story about the hero's journey—a person who goes out into the world, faces a crisis, conquers a threat, and returns home a changed person. Think of *Lord of the Rings* or *Harry Potter*, stories I have devoured and loved. Threads of this narrative structure are found everywhere in religion, literature, politics, and the media. The hero's journey is about conquering the self, destroying the ego, and gathering new knowledge. We have told this story over and over until it has become deeply integrated into our culture and shaped who we believe we are as individuals and how we face adversity. In part, I think this is why much of the mental health conversation is about the individual rather than the ways that person has been shaped by the world around her.

This book has told different kinds of stories. My path to healing did not take place in a vacuum, where I alone came to defeat the enemy that was mental illness. I haven't scaled or conquered or overthrown anything. My journey has instead been an un-education—a deep dive into the biology of mental illness, the stories I have been fed, and the realization that my own knowledge and strength are essential tools in my healing. I have learned to accept the gift of my body, my mind, and the sacredness of my whole self in connection with others. My story isn't a hero's journey, but it is the bravest thing I have ever done.

EPILOGUE

THERE ARE TINY SLIVERS of time in our lives when we experience moments of clarity, truth, and peace. We search and search for patterns in the infinite randomness and uncertainty of life, never allowing ourselves to admit that nothing is really under our control. So, when the light of knowledge does shine down for one startling moment, we sit up and take notice.

One of those times came for me on a long and boring drive from Toronto to my home in Ottawa; what was supposed to have been a fun weekend away was full of insomnia and fear. I was deep into another relapse of anxiety, impatient and frustrated with myself that I would never "get over" this illness. It had been almost two decades since my teenage crisis, and while my life was full of joy and beauty, I couldn't shake the shadows.

I turned on the radio to keep myself awake and listened to a program called *Tapestry*, which explores spirituality, religion, and the meaning of life. It was a rebroadcast of an older interview with the Irish poet John O'Donohue, who quoted Meister Eckhart (a fourteenth-century German mystic): "There is a place in the soul that neither time nor space nor no created thing can touch." O'Donohue went on to ask listeners, "What if I told you that you're not broken? What if I told you that there is a place inside you that no one has ever reached or hurt or damaged—a place where there is peace, serenity, courage, and healing; that at your deepest core you don't actually belong to yourself but to a beauty, an intimacy, and a shelter that offers you every freedom you could imagine."[1]

I finished the radio program, made it home safely, and in the days and weeks that followed, I pondered the answer to O'Donohue's question: *What if I told you that you're not broken?*

I decided to find out. And the answer to that question is this book.

The first thing I needed to understand was who told me I was broken in the first place. I read about the history of hysteria, the construct of mental illness as a female disease, the early categorization of symptoms and the creation of the DSM, sex differences for biological risk factors of mental illness, and the neuroscientific understanding of emotions. I learned that emotions aren't triggered, they are *created*. I realized that we still don't understand what makes a mind, and that the mystery and sacredness of that was something I valued. I learned that my brain is wired for survival, and that other brains can be both good and bad for me, in that my body can be regulated or stressed by other people. I began to practice embodiment and explored how I had internalized social and cultural messages about my body. I studied books about patriarchy, colonialism, and white-body supremacy.

I started to tell myself that I wasn't broken. I unraveled our cultural stories of health and disease and found that they were untrue or at least deeply flawed. I discovered there *was* a place deep inside me where I was free, where I was not defined by mental illness, where I was a whole person worthy of goodness and love. Pain and suffering still came, but I met them with more respect and reverence for what they were able to teach me, rather than what they would *do* to me.

Part of this process, I know, was the gift of time and wisdom. I look back at my younger self and wonder how she would have evolved if she had been able to see those social forces at work; if she had been taught to say no, to say "This doesn't work for me." Would she have discovered the freedom to write a different story about her life?

My grandmother never got the opportunity to rewrite her own story. I feel now that I hold all the joy and despair of her life within me, not as a piece of genetic misfortune but as a touchstone for my own pain and happiness. My grandmother loved and lived in an expansive and passionate way, and though the illness she faced (and the treatment she received) took away her freedom, I don't think it could have ever stripped her of her human dignity or her ability to love and be loved in return. I hope I have done justice to her story, and I feel a deep sense of gratitude for her role in my life.

THERE IS NO CURE for mental illness, but there can be healing.

If we return to the analogy of the river, we see that women continue to be pushed into the water because of sexism, racism, oppression, poverty, and violence—all deeply embedded in our social systems. Therapists and family members pull people to safety, or we throw the life raft of medication to those who need it.[2] Tragically, some women drown along the way.

To better care for women, we need both prevention *and* intervention. We need to stop pushing women into the water, and we also need to provide a range of supports that are appropriate for each individual, rather than the standard that's been developed from biased knowledge about white cisgender nondisabled men.

I've been pulled out of that river by wonderful therapists, and I've also spent time on my medication raft when needed. But healing didn't begin for me until I learned how to swim, until I got strong enough that I was able to pull *myself* over to the river's edge. This has not prevented me from being thrown back into the water, but each time, I find myself stronger than I was before.

Women's pain and suffering is not all in our heads. It's in our brains, our minds, and our bodies; it's also in the brains, minds, and bodies of other human beings. It trickles in from the social, economic, and political world in which we live, and it is woven into the cultural story of our lives. To recover from this is to acknowledge that we all contribute to this pain and that we all have a responsibility to heal.

ACKNOWLEDGMENTS

THIS BOOK NEVER would have been written without my teacher and mentor Ann Douglas, whom I thank for her expert guidance and unwavering support through the proposal writing experience. Ann also deserves full credit for the superb title of this book.

To all the folks at Greystone Books, who took their chances with a fledgling author and made me feel so welcome and supported. My sincere gratitude to Jennifer Croll and Jen Gauthier for believing in this book. I especially owe so much to my editor extraordinaire Paula Ayer, who took an unwieldy first draft and helped me turn it into something much clearer and vastly improved. Thank you to Crissy Calhoun, who handled the later stages of editing with such expertise, and to my proofreader, Dawn Loewen, for her care and skill. To Belle Wuthrich: I couldn't have asked for a more beautiful cover design that represents women's power and pain in equal measure. To my fact-checker Emily Latimer, whose precision and thoroughness were a gift.

A heartfelt thank-you to my writing tribe, who was with me for the earlier stages of this book: Trina, Jane, Pamela, Maggie, and Kaitlin, for sharing your own beautiful writing with me and allowing me to share mine. And to the teachers and participants in my University of King's College writing workshops, thank you for your comments on the first chapter. Your insights have been instrumental in the writing of this book. A special thanks goes out to Trina Warner and Lilly Bianchi, who read every word of the initial draft and provided me with such valuable feedback.

To all the women who took part in this book, thank you. Your stories have changed me, your hard work has inspired me, and I hope that what you see in these pages is an accurate reflection of your strength and perseverance. You are true heroes. Special thanks to Elizabeth Tobin for your detailed and stunning artwork of the process of neurotransmission. Deep gratitude and thanks to my therapist, Rebecca Minish, who was with me from the early days of this book and who taught me how to truly live in my body.

To my parents, Nick and Sharleen. Thank you for raising me to be curious, passionate, and only slightly obsessive. Many people with mental illness do not have family support, and I am forever grateful that you intervened all those years ago and got me the help I needed. Thank you, too, to my brother Mike, who provides unwavering support for my (many) passion projects.

To my life partner and friend, Tom Stacey: I definitely could not have written this book without you. For all the times I wailed "I can't do this!" thank you for patiently guiding me back to my desk. Thank you to my daughters for your support and understanding while I missed a lot of family time to work on this book, and for cheering me on.

Finally, to Kit. I wish so much that you were here to see the publication of this book. Thank you for showing me the truth of what it means to be a woman in this world—I will forever cherish my box full of darkness, and I continue to discover all the places where the light shines through.

NOTES

Introduction

1 Ronald C. Kessler et al., "Lifetime Prevalence and Age-of-Onset Distributions of *DSM-IV* Disorders in the National Comorbidity Survey Replication," *Archives of General Psychiatry* 62, no. 6 (June 2005): 593–602, doi.org/10.1001/archpsyc.62.6.593.

2 J. Breslau et al., "Sex Differences in Recent First-Onset Depression in an Epidemiological Sample of Adolescents," *Translational Psychiatry* 7, no. 5 (May 2017): e1139, doi.org/10.1038/tp.2017.105.

3 Sarah-Jayne Blakemore, "Adolescence and Mental Health," *The Lancet* 393, no. 10185 (May 18, 2019): 2030–31, doi.org/10.1016/s0140-6736(19)31013-x.

4 Lisa Feldman Barrett, *Seven and a Half Lessons About the Brain* (New York: Mariner Books, 2020), 74–77.

5 World Health Organization, "Gender and Mental Health," WHO Department of Gender and Women's Health, June 2002, apps.who.int/iris/handle/10665/68884.

6 Etienne G. Krug et al., eds., *World Report on Violence and Health* (Geneva: World Health Organization, 2002), apps.who.int/iris/bitstream/handle/10665/42495/9241545615_eng.pdf.

7 Laura Savage, "Intimate Partner Violence: Experiences of Young Women in Canada, 2018," Statistics Canada, May 19, 2021, www150.statcan.gc.ca/n1/pub/85-002-x/2021001/article/00009-eng.htm.

8 Giussy Barbara et al., "Characteristics of Sexual Violence Against Adolescent Girls: A 10 Years' Retrospective Study of 731 Sexually Abused Adolescents," *International Journal of Women's Health* 14 (2022): 311–21, doi.org/10.2147/IJWH.S343935.

9 Cecilia Tasca, Mariangela Rapetti, Mauro G. Carta, and Bianca Fadda, "Women and Hysteria in the History of Mental Health," *Clinical Practice & Epidemiology in Mental Health* 8 (2012): 110–19, doi.org/10.2174/1745017901208010110.

10 Lauren Slater, *Blue Dreams: The Science and the Story of the Drugs That Changed Our Minds* (New York: Little Brown and Company, 2018), 163.

11 Joanna Moncrieff et al., "The Serotonin Theory of Depression: A Systematic Umbrella Review of the Evidence," *Molecular Psychiatry* 27, no. 7 (July 2022): 1–14, doi.org/10.1038/s41380-022-01661-0.

12   World Health Organization, "Gender and Mental Health."

13   Damian F. Santomauro et al., "Global Prevalence and Burden of Depressive and Anxiety Disorders in 204 Countries and Territories in 2020 Due to the COVID-19 Pandemic," *The Lancet* 398, no. 10312 (November 6, 2021): 1700–1712, doi.org/10.1016/S0140-6736(21)02143-7.

14   Kristen L. Syme and Edward H. Hagen, "Mental Health Is Biological Health: Why Tackling 'Diseases of the Mind' Is an Imperative for Biological Anthropology in the 21st Century," *American Journal of Biological Anthropology* 171, no. S70 (May 2020): 87–117, doi.org/10.1002/ajpa.23965.

15   Ana Sabela Álvarez, Marco Pagani, and Paolo Meucci, "The Clinical Application of the Biopsychosocial Model in Mental Health: A Research Critique," *American Journal of Physical Medicine & Rehabilitation* 91, no. 13 (February 2012): S173–80, doi.org/10.1097/PHM.0b013e31823d54be.

16   George L. Engel, "The Biopsychosocial Model and the Education of Health Professionals," *Annals of the New York Academy of Sciences* 310, no. 1 (June 1978): 169–81, doi.org/10.1111/j.1749-6632.1978.tb22070.x.

17   Andrew J. Hogan, "Social and Medical Models of Disability and Mental Health: Evolution and Renewal," *Canadian Medical Association Journal* 191, no. 1 (January 7, 2019): E16–18, doi.org/10.1503/cmaj.181008.

18   Álvarez, Pagani, and Meucci, "The Clinical Application of the Biopsychosocial Model."

19   Ilyas Sagar-Ouriaghli et al., "Improving Mental Health Service Utilization Among Men: A Systematic Review and Synthesis of Behavior Change Techniques Within Interventions Targeting Help-Seeking," *American Journal of Men's Health* 13, no. 3 (May–June 2019), doi.org/10.1177/1557988319857009.

20   Donna Tedstone Doherty and Yulia Kartalova-O'Doherty, "Gender and Self-Reported Mental Health Problems: Predictors of Help Seeking From a General Practitioner," *British Journal of Health Psychology* 15, no. 1 (February 2010): 213–28, doi.org/10.1348/135910709X457423.

1: Hysteria in Action

1   Harriet A. Washington, *Infectious Madness: The Surprising Science of How We "Catch" Mental Illness* (New York: Little Brown and Company, 2015), 12.

2   Lisa Mosconi, *The XX Brain: The Groundbreaking Science Empowering Women to Maximize Cognitive Health and Prevent Alzheimer's Disease* (New York: Avery, 2020), 11.

3   E. W. Freeman, "Associations of Depression With the Transition to Menopause," *Menopause* 17, no. 4 (July 2010): 823–27, doi.org/10.1097/gme.0b013e3181db9f8b.

4   S. Nassir Ghaemi and Shannon Dalley, "The Bipolar Spectrum: Conceptions and Misconceptions," *Australian & New Zealand Journal of Psychiatry* 48, no. 4 (April 2014): 314–24, doi.org/10.1177/0004867413504830.

5 Seyed Mehdi Samimi Ardestani et al., "Bipolar Spectrum in Patients With Conversion Disorder," *Iranian Journal of Psychiatry and Behavioral Sciences* 14, no. 4 (September 2020), doi.org/10.5812/ijpbs.107466.

6 Mosconi, *The xx Brain*, 16–18.

7 National Institutes of Health, "Conversion Disorder," Genetic and Rare Diseases Information Center (GARD), accessed October 14, 2021, rarediseases. info.nih.gov/diseases/6191/conversion-disorder.

8 Shahid Ali et al., "Conversion Disorder—Mind Versus Body: A Review," *Innovations in Clinical Neuroscience* 12, no. 5–6 (June 2015): 27–33, ncbi.nlm. nih.gov/pmc/articles/PMC4479361.

9 Anne Harrington, "A Tale of Two Disorders: Syphilis, Hysteria and the Struggle to Treat Mental Illness," *Nature* 572 (August 2019): 436–37, doi.org/10.1038/d41586-019-02476-w.

10 Ali et al., "Conversion Disorder."

11 Allan H. Ropper and Brian David Burrell, *How the Brain Lost Its Mind: Sex, Hysteria, and the Riddle of Mental Illness* (New York: Avery, 2019), 47.

12 *Jean-Martin Charcot Demonstrating Hysteria in a Hypnotised Patient at the Salpêtrière.* Etching by A. Lurat, 1888, after P.A.A. Brouillet, 1887. Wellcome Collection. Attribution 4.0 International (CC BY 4.0). wellcomecollection.org/works/qrkb3myu.

13 Harvard Health Publishing, "Conversion Disorder," March 9, 2014, health. harvard.edu/newsletter_article/Conversion_disorder.

14 Elinor Cleghorn, *Unwell Women: Misdiagnosis and Myth in a Man-Made World* (New York: Dutton, 2021), 28.

15 Peter T. Leeson and Jacob W. Russ, "Witch Trials," *Economic Journal* 128, no. 613 (August 2018): 2066–105, doi.org/10.1111/ecoj.12498.

16 G. S. Rousseau, "'A Strange Pathology': Hysteria in the Early Modern World, 1500–1800," in *Hysteria Beyond Freud*, authored by Sander L. Gilman et al. (Berkeley: University of California Press, 1993), 97.

17 Barbara Ehrenreich and Deirdre English, *Witches, Midwives, and Nurses: A History of Women Healers*, 2nd ed. (New York City: The Feminist Press at CUNY, 2010), 31–33. This book has been criticized for exaggerating the number of midwives among the convicted witches and for misrepresenting the religious identity of most lay healers. (They likely did not gather in covens or engage in pagan rituals; they were likely practicing Christians.) In a revised edition, Ehrenreich and English stand by their assertion that male physicians benefited from suppressing female lay healers and early female physicians.

18 Mark S. Micale, *Approaching Hysteria* (Princeton, NJ: Princeton University Press, 2019), 20.

19 Ehrenreich and English, *Witches, Midwives, and Nurses*, 39.

20 Cleghorn, *Unwell Women*, 45.

21 Edward Jorden, *A Briefe Discourse of a Disease Called the Suffocation of the Mother* (London: John Windet, 1603), books.google.co.uk/books?id=6ZIPAQAAIAAJ; British

Library, "First English Book on Hysteria, 1603," accessed July 25, 2023, bl.uk/collection-items/first-english-book-on-hysteria-1603.

22   Cleghorn, *Unwell Women*, 46.

23   Maya Dusenbery, *Doing Harm: The Truth About How Bad Medicine and Lazy Science Leave Women Dismissed, Misdiagnosed, and Sick* (New York: Harper Collins, 2018), 65.

24   Heather Meek, "Medical Men, Women of Letters, and Treatments for Eighteenth-Century Hysteria," *Journal of Medical Humanities* 34, no. 1 (March 2013): 1–14, doi.org/10.1007/s10912-012-9194-4.

25   Ropper and Burrell, *How the Brain Lost Its Mind*, 52.

26   Neeta Mehta, "Mind-Body Dualism: A Critique From a Health Perspective," *Mens Sana Monographs* 9, no. 1 (2011): 202–9, ncbi.nlm.nih.gov/pmc/articles/PMC3115289/.

27   Ada McVean, "The History of Hysteria," McGill Office for Science and Society, July 31, 2017, mcgill.ca/oss/article/history-quackery/history-hysteria.

28   Charles Darwin, *The Descent of Man, and Selection in Relation to Sex* (London: John Murray, 1871), 327.

29   Angela Saini, *Inferior: How Science Got Women Wrong—and the New Research That's Rewriting the Story* (Boston: Beacon Press, 2017), 14.

30   Micale, *Approaching Hysteria*, 285.

2: Gender Bias in Mental Health Care

1   Caroline Criado Perez, *Invisible Women: Data Bias in a World Designed for Men* (New York: Abrams Press, 2019), 318.

2   Perez, *Invisible Women*, 196.

3   Megan Brenan, "40% of Americans Believe in Creationism," Gallup, July 26, 2019, news.gallup.com/poll/261680/americans-believe-creationism.aspx; Pamela Milne, "Genesis From Eve's Point of View," *Washington Post*, March 26, 1989, washingtonpost.com/archive/opinions/1989/03/26/genesis-from-eves-point-of-view/dc371184-1f4c-4142-ac2d-d5efee72a0da.

4   Jean-Baptiste Bonnard, "Male and Female Bodies According to Ancient Greek Physicians," *Clio* 37 (2013), doi.org/10.4000/cliowgh.339.

5   Katrina Hui et al., "Recognizing and Addressing Implicit Gender Bias in Medicine," *Canadian Medical Association Journal* 192, no. 42 (October 2020): E1269–70, doi.org/10.1503/cmaj.200286.

6   Amy Westervelt, "The Medical Research Gender Gap: How Excluding Women From Clinical Trials Is Hurting Our Health," *The Guardian*, April 30, 2015, theguardian.com/lifeandstyle/2015/apr/30/fda-clinical-trials-gender-gap-epa-nih-institute-of-medicine-cardiovascular-disease.

7   Natalie. A. DiPietro Mager and Katherine A. Liu, "Women's Involvement in Clinical Trials: Historical Perspective and Future Implications," *Pharmacy Practice* (Granada) 14, no. 1 (March 2016): 708, doi.org/10.18549/PharmPract.2016.01.708.

8 Irving Zucker and Brian J. Prendergast, "Sex Differences in Pharmacokinetics Predict Adverse Drug Reactions in Women," *Biology of Sex Differences* 11, no. 1 (June 2020): 32, doi.org/10.1186/s13293-020-00308-5.

9 T. K. Sundari Ravindran, "Making Pharmaceutical Research and Regulation Work for Women," *BMJ* 371 (October 2020): m3808, doi.org/10.1136/bmj.m3808.

10 Ann-Marie G. de Lange, Emily G. Jacobs, and Liisa A. M. Galea, "The Scientific Body of Knowledge: Whose Body Does It Serve? A Spotlight on Women's Brain Health," *Frontiers in Neuroendocrinology* 60 (January 2021): 100898, doi.org/10.1016/j.yfrne.2020.100898.

11 European Commission, "Gender Equality in Research and Innovation," *Strategic Plan 2020–2024*, research-and-innovation.ec.europa.eu/strategy/strategy-2020-2024/democracy-and-rights/gender-equality-research-and-innovation_en.

12 Philippe Kerr et al., "Allostatic Load and Women's Brain Health: A Systematic Review," *Frontiers in Neuroendocrinology* 59 (October 2020): 100858, doi.org/10.1016/j.yfrne.2020.100858.

13 World Health Organization, "Gender," accessed October 14, 2021, who.int/westernpacific/health-topics/gender.

14 Emma Beddington, "The Zoologist Sticking Her Neck Out in the Battle of the Sexes," *The Guardian*, March 6, 2022, theguardian.com/science/2022/mar/06/the-zoologist-sticking-her-neck-out-in-the-battle-of-the-sexes.

15 Rand S. Eid, Aarthi R. Gobinath, and Liisa A. M. Galea, "Sex Differences in Depression: Insights From Clinical and Preclinical Studies," *Progress in Neurobiology* 176 (May 2019): 86–102, doi.org/10.1016/j.pneurobio.2019.01.006.

16 Elinor Cleghorn, *Unwell Women: Misdiagnosis and Myth in a Man-Made World* (New York: Dutton, 2021), 2.

17 Lorraine Greaves and Stacey A. Ritz, "Sex, Gender and Health: Mapping the Landscape of Research and Policy," *International Journal of Environmental Research and Public Health* 19, no. 5 (February 2022): 2563, doi.org/10.3390/ijerph19052563.

18 Rebecca K. Rechlin et al., "Harnessing the Power of Sex Differences: What a Difference Ten Years Did Not Make," *bioRxiv*, November 4, 2021, doi.org/10.1101/2021.06.30.450396.

19 David J. Greenblatt, Jerold S. Harmatz, and Thomas Roth, "Zolpidem and Gender: Are Women Really at Risk?," *Journal of Clinical Psychopharmacology* 39, no. 3 (June 2019): 189–99, doi.org/10.1097/JCP.0000000000001026.

20 Greenblatt, Harmatz, and Roth, "Zolpidem and Gender."

21 Eid, Gobinath, and Galea, "Sex Differences in Depression"; Evelyn Bromet et al., "Cross-National Epidemiology of DSM-IV Major Depressive Episode," *BMC Medicine* 9 (July 2011): 90, doi.org/10.1186/1741-7015-9-90.

22 Ying Sun et al., "Comparison of Mental Health Symptoms Before and During the COVID-19 Pandemic: Evidence From a Systematic Review and Meta-Analysis of 134 Cohorts," *BMJ* 380 (March 2023): e074224, doi.org/10.1136/bmj-2022-074224.

23 Nirmita Panchal, Heather Saunders, Robin Rudowitz, and Cynthia Cox, "The Implications of COVID-19 for Mental Health and Substance Use," KFF, March 20, 2023, kff.org/coronavirus-covid-19/issue-brief/the-implications-of-covid-19-for-mental-health-and-substance-use.

24 Christine Kuehner, "Why Is Depression More Common Among Women Than Among Men?," *The Lancet Psychiatry* 4, no. 2 (February 2017): 146–58, doi.org/10.1016/S2215-0366(16)30263-2.

25 Londa Schiebinger, "Women's Health and Clinical Trials," *Journal of Clinical Investigation* 112, no. 7 (October 2003): 973–77, doi.org/10.1172/JCI19993; Zucker and Prendergast, "Sex Differences in Pharmacokinetics."

26 Perez, *Invisible Women*, 204; Louise M. Howard, Anna M. Ehrlich, Freya Gamlen, and Sian Oram, "Gender-Neutral Mental Health Research Is Sex and Gender Biased," *The Lancet Psychiatry* 4, no. 1 (January 2017): 9–11, doi.org/10.1016/S2215-0366(16)30209-7; Institute of Medicine (US) Board on Health Sciences Policy, *Inclusion of Women in Clinical Trials: Policies for Population Subgroups* (1993), ncbi.nlm.nih.gov/books/NBK221285.

27 Tara Haelle, "Lack of Data on COVID-19 Vaccines and Periods Inspired Two Feminist Scientists to Learn More," *Elemental* (blog), April 12, 2021, elemental.medium.com/lack-of-data-on-covid-19-vaccines-and-periods-inspired-two-feminist-scientists-to-learn-more-b4c29395fb5.

28 Alison Edelman et al., "Association Between Menstrual Cycle Length and COVID-19 Vaccination: Global, Retrospective Cohort Study of Prospectively Collected Data," *BMJ Medicine* 1, no. 1 (September 2022): e000297, doi.org/10.1136/bmjmed-2022-000297.

29 Amaia Bacigalupe and Unai Martín, "Gender Inequalities in Depression/Anxiety and the Consumption of Psychotropic Drugs: Are We Medicalising Women's Mental Health?," *Scandinavian Journal of Public Health* 49, no. 3 (May 2021): 317–24, doi.org/10.1177/1403494820944736.

30 Maureen C. McHugh and Joan C. Chrisler, eds., *The Wrong Prescription for Women: How Medicine and Media Create a "Need" for Treatments, Drugs, and Surgery* (Santa Barbara, CA: Praeger, 2015), 2–3.

31 Dena T. Smith, Dawne M. Mouzon, and Marta Elliott, "Reviewing the Assumptions About Men's Mental Health: An Exploration of the Gender Binary," *American Journal of Men's Health* 12, no. 1 (January 2018): 78–89, doi.org/10.1177/1557988316630953.

32 Bacigalupe and Martín, "Gender Inequalities in Depression/Anxiety."

33 Lisa Feldman Barrett, "The Theory of Constructed Emotion: An Active Inference Account of Interoception and Categorization," *Social Cognitive and Affective Neuroscience* 12, no. 1 (January 1, 2017): 1–23, doi.org/10.1093/scan/nsw154.

34 National Institute of Mental Health, "Depression," accessed July 1, 2023, nimh.nih.gov/health/topics/depression.

35 Christine D. Wilson-Mendenhall, Lisa Feldman Barrett, and Lawrence W. Barsalou, "Situating Emotional Experience," *Frontiers in Human Neuroscience* 7 (November 2013): 764, doi.org/10.3389/fnhum.2013.00764.

36   Lisa Feldman Barrett, Lucy Robin, Paula R. Pietromonaco, and Kristen M. Eyssell, "Are Women the 'More Emotional' Sex? Evidence From Emotional Experiences in Social Context," *Cognition and Emotion* 12, no. 4 (1998): 555–78, doi.org/10.1080/026999398379565.

37   Lisa Feldman Barrett, "Myth of the Male Brain vs. the Female Brain," *How Emotions Are Made* (New York: Houghton Mifflin Harcourt, 2017), ch11n17, accessed November 4, 2021, how-emotions-are-made.com/notes/Myth_of_ the_male_brain_vs._the_female_brain.

38   Dr. Sarah McKay, *The Women's Brain Book: The Neuroscience of Health, Hormones, and Happiness* (Sydney: Hachette Australia, 2018), 94–99.

39   Jane Ussher, "The Myth of Premenstrual Moodiness," *The Conversation*, December 11, 2012, theconversation.com/the-myth-of-premenstrual-moodiness-10289.

40   Sally King, "Premenstrual Syndrome (PMS) and the Myth of the Irrational Female," in *The Palgrave Handbook of Critical Menstruation Studies*, eds. C. Bobel et al. (Singapore: Palgrave Macmillan, 2020), ncbi.nlm.nih.gov/books/NBK565629.

41   Tory A. Eisenlohr-Moul, "Commentary on Joyce et al.: Studying Menstrual Cycle Effects on Behavior Requires Within-Person Designs and Attention to Individual Differences in Hormone Sensitivity," *Addiction* 116, no. 10 (October 2021): 2759–60, doi.org/10.1111/add.15576.

42   David P. Schmitt, "Are Women More Emotional Than Men?," *Psychology Today* April 10, 2015, psychologytoday.com/ca/blog/sexual-personalities/201504/ are-women-more-emotional-men.

43   Schmitt, "Are Women More Emotional Than Men?"

44   E. Ashby Plant, Janet Shibley Hyde, Dacher Keltner, and Patricia G. Devine, "The Gender Stereotyping of Emotions," *Psychology of Women Quarterly* 24, no. 1 (March 2000): 81–92, doi.org/10.1111/j.1471-6402.2000.tb01024.x.

45   Lisa Feldman Barrett, "That Is Not How Your Brain Works," *Nautilus*, March 3, 2021, nautil.us/that-is-not-how-your-brain-works-238138.

3: Biology, Hormones, and Mental Health

1   Jane Austen, *Persuasion* (Everyman's Library: Alfred A. Knopf, 1996), 231.

2   National Institutes of Health, "Common Genetic Factors Found in 5 Mental Disorders," *NIH Research Matters*, March 18, 2013, www.nih.gov/news-events/ nih-research-matters/common-genetic-factors-found-5-mental-disorders.

3   Gretchen Livingston, "They're Waiting Longer, but U.S. Women Today More Likely to Have Children Than a Decade Ago," Pew Research Center, January 18, 2018, pewresearch.org/social-trends/2018/01/18/theyre-waiting-longer-but-u-s-women-today-more-likely-to-have-children-than-a-decade-ago.

4   Sophie Schweizer-Schubert et al., "Steroid Hormone Sensitivity in Reproductive Mood Disorders: On the Role of the $GABA_A$ Receptor Complex and Stress During Hormonal Transitions," *Frontiers in Medicine* 7 (January 2021), doi.org/10.3389/fmed.2020.479646.

5   Vivien K. Burt and Kira Stein, "Epidemiology of Depression Throughout the Female Life Cycle," *Journal of Clinical Psychiatry* 63, suppl. 7 (2002): 9–15, pubmed.ncbi.nlm.nih.gov/11995779.

6   Lisa Mosconi et al., "Menopause Impacts Human Brain Structure, Connectivity, Energy Metabolism, and Amyloid-Beta Deposition," *Scientific Reports* 11 (June 2021): 10867, doi.org/10.1038/s41598-021-90084-y.

7   Cheryl L. Sisk and Douglas L. Foster, "The Neural Basis of Puberty and Adolescence," *Nature Neuroscience* 7 (October 2004): 1040–47, doi.org/10.1038/nn1326.

8   Dr. Sarah McKay, *The Women's Brain Book: The Neuroscience of Health, Hormones, and Happiness* (Sydney: Hachette Australia, 2018).

9   Dr. Jen Gunter, *The Menopause Manifesto: Own Your Health With Facts and Feminism* (Toronto: Penguin Random House Canada, 2021).

10   McKay, *The Women's Brain Book*, 23–24.

11   Gunter, *The Menopause Manifesto*, 149.

12   Paul Andrews and Jay Amsterdam, "A Hormetic Approach to Understanding Antidepressant Effectiveness and the Development of Antidepressant Tolerance—a Conceptual View," *Psychiatria Polska* 54, no. 6 (December 2020): 1067–90, doi.org/10.12740/PP/120084.

13   Andrée-Anne Hudon Thibeault, J. Thomas Sanderson, and Cathy Vaillancourt, "Serotonin-Estrogen Interactions: What Can We Learn from Pregnancy?," *Biochimie* 161 (June 2019): 88–108, doi.org/10.1016/j.biochi.2019.03.023.

14   McKay, *The Women's Brain Book*, 110.

15   Elseline Hoekzema et al., "Pregnancy Leads to Long-Lasting Changes in Human Brain Structure," *Nature Neuroscience* 20 (February 2017): 287–96, doi.org/10.1038/nn.4458.

16   Mosconi et al., "Menopause Impacts Human Brain Structure."

17   Centers for Disease Control and Prevention, "Data and Statistics on Children's Mental Health," Centers for Disease Control and Prevention, accessed June 15, 2020, cdc.gov/childrensmentalhealth/data.html.

18   Nicole Racine et al., "Global Prevalence of Depressive and Anxiety Symptoms in Children and Adolescents During COVID-19: A Meta-Analysis," *JAMA Pediatrics* 175, no. 11 (August 2021): 1142–50, doi.org/10.1001/jamapediatrics.2021.2482.

19   Denis Campbell, "Stress and Social Media Fuel Mental Health Crisis Among Girls," *The Guardian*, September 23, 2017, theguardian.com/society/2017/sep/23/stress-anxiety-fuel-mental-health-crisis-girls-young-women.

20   Tamsin Newlove-Delgado et al., "Mental Health of Children and Young People in England, 2021: Wave 2 Follow Up to the 2017 Survey," National Health Service (NHS) Digital, September 30, 2021, digital.nhs.uk/data-and-information/publications/statistical/mental-health-of-children-and-young-people-in-england/2021-follow-up-to-the-2017-survey.

21   William Bor, Angela J. Dean, Jacob Najman, and Reza Hayatbakhsh, "Are Child and Adolescent Mental Health Problems Increasing in the 21st Century?

A Systematic Review," *Australian & New Zealand Journal of Psychiatry* 48, no. 7 (July 2014): 606–16, doi.org/10.1177/0004867414533834.

22 Rachel H. B. Mitchell et al., "Sex Differences in Suicide Trends Among Adolescents Aged 10 to 14 Years in Canada," *Canadian Journal of Psychiatry* 68, no. 7 (July 2023): 547–49, doi.org/10.1177/07067437231173370.

23 Lisa Eiland and Russell D. Romeo, "Stress and the Developing Adolescent Brain," *Neuroscience* 249 (September 2013): 162–71, doi.org/10.1016/j.neuroscience.2012.10.048.

24 Russell D. Romeo, "The Teenage Brain: The Stress Response and the Adolescent Brain," *Current Directions in Psychological Science* 22, no. 2 (April 2013): 140–45, doi.org/10.1177/0963721413475445.

25 Alaine E. Reschke-Hernández, Katrina L. Okerstrom, Angela Bowles Edwards, and Daniel Tranel, "Sex and Stress: Men and Women Show Different Cortisol Responses to Psychological Stress Induced by the Trier Social Stress Test and the Iowa Singing Social Stress Test," *Journal of Neuroscience Research* 95, no. 1–2 (January/February 2017): 106–14, doi.org/10.1002/jnr.23851.

26 Rohit Verma, Yatan Pal Singh Balhara, and Chandra Shekhar Gupta, "Gender Differences in Stress Response: Role of Developmental and Biological Determinants," *Industrial Psychiatry Journal* 20, no. 1 (January–June 2011): 4–10, doi.org/10.4103/0972-6748.98407.

27 Rebecca Greenfield, "Sexism at Facebook Is What Made It Facebook," *The Atlantic*, July 6, 2012, theatlantic.com/technology/archive/2012/07/sexism-facebook-what-made-it-facebook/326191.

28 Johann Hari, *Stolen Focus: Why You Can't Pay Attention—and How to Think Deeply Again* (New York: Crown, 2022).

29 Yvonne Kelly, Afshin Zilanawala, Cara Booker, and Amanda Sacker, "Social Media Use and Adolescent Mental Health: Findings From the UK Millennium Cohort Study," *eClinicalMedicine* 6 (December 2018): 59–68, doi.org/10.1016/j.eclinm.2018.12.005.

30 Leslie Morrison Gutman and Natasha Codiroli McMaster, "Gendered Pathways of Internalizing Problems From Early Childhood to Adolescence and Associated Adolescent Outcomes," *Journal of Abnormal Child Psychology* 48 (May 2020): 703–18, doi.org/10.1007/s10802-020-00623-w.

31 Donna Jackson Nakazawa, *Girls on the Brink: Helping Our Daughters Thrive in an Era of Increased Anxiety, Depression, and Social Media* (New York: Harmony, 2022), 69.

32 Jonathon Novello, "The Seven Tasks of Adolescence: Task 2—Joining a New Tribe," Michigan State University Health 4U Program, September 12, 2017, health4u.msu.edu/articles/2017-the-seven-tasks-of-adolescence-task-2-joining-a-new-tribe.

33 Russell M. Viner et al., "Roles of Cyberbullying, Sleep, and Physical Activity in Mediating the Effects of Social Media Use on Mental Health and Wellbeing Among Young People in England: A Secondary Analysis of Longitudinal Data," *The Lancet Child & Adolescent Health* 3, no. 10 (October 2019): 685–96, doi.org/10.1016/S2352-4642(19)30186-5.

34 Viner et al., "Roles of Cyberbullying."

35 Aja Romano, "Pixar's *Turning Red* Is an Unlikely Culture War Battleground," *Vox*, March 17, 2022, vox.com/culture/22981394/turning-red-reviews-controversy-reactions-parents.

36 UC San Diego Center on Gender Equity and Health, *Measuring #MeToo: A National Study on Sexual Harassment and Assault*, April 2019, stopstreetharassment.org/wp-content/uploads/2012/08/2019-MeToo-National-Sexual-Harassment-and-Assault-Report.pdf.

37 Sophie Khadr et al., "Mental and Sexual Health Outcomes Following Sexual Assault in Adolescents: A Prospective Cohort Study," *The Lancet Child & Adolescent Health* 2, no. 9 (September 2018): 654–65, doi.org/10.1016/S2352-4642(18)30202-5.

38 Andy Fell, "Hippocampus Is the Brain's Storyteller," UC Davis, September 29, 2021, ucdavis.edu/health/news/hippocampus-brains-storyteller.

39 Krystin Arneson, "Why Doesn't the US Have Mandated Paid Maternity Leave?," June 28, 2021, bbc.com/worklife/article/20210624-why-doesnt-the-us-have-mandated-paid-maternity-leave.

40 Andrea Doucet, Sophie Mathieu, and Lindsey McKay, "Redesign Parental Leave System to Enhance Gender Equality," *Policy Options*, October 27, 2020, policyoptions.irpp.org/magazines/october-2020/redesign-parental-leave-system-to-enhance-gender-equality.

41 Kristen Schultz Lee and Hiroshi Ono, "Paid Family Leave Makes People Happier, Global Data Shows," *The Conversation*, April 6, 2022, theconversation.com/paid-family-leave-makes-people-happier-global-data-shows-179539.

42 Andrea Lawson et al., "The Relationship Between Sleep and Postpartum Mental Disorders: A Systematic Review," *Journal of Affective Disorders* 176 (May 2015): 65–77, doi.org/10.1016/j.jad.2015.01.017.

43 Cindy-Lee Dennis et al., "Traditional Postpartum Practices and Rituals: A Qualitative Systematic Review," *Women's Health* 3, no. 4 (July 2007): 487–502, doi.org/10.2217/17455057.3.4.487.

44 Miriam T. Weber, Pauline M. Maki, and Michael P. McDermott, "Cognition and Mood in Perimenopause: A Systematic Review and Meta-Analysis," *Journal of Steroid Biochemistry and Molecular Biology* 142 (July 2014): 90–98, doi.org/10.1016/j.jsbmb.2013.06.001.

45 Gunter, *The Menopause Manifesto*, x.

46 Weber, Maki, and McDermott, "Cognition and Mood in Perimenopause."

47 Gunter, *The Menopause Manifesto*, 154.

48 McKay, *The Women's Brain Book*, 222.

49 McKay, *The Women's Brain Book*, 232.

50 McKay, *The Women's Brain Book*, 232.

51 Angelo Cagnacci and Martina Venier, "The Controversial History of Hormone Replacement Therapy," *Medicina* 55, no. 9 (September 2019): 602, doi.org/10.3390/medicina55090602.

52 Jayashri Kulkarni, "There's No 'Rushing Women's Syndrome' but Hormones Affect Mental Health," *The Conversation*, June 20, 2014, theconversation.com/theres-no-rushing-womens-syndrome-but-hormones-affect-mental-health-28136.

53 Sabrina Faleschini et al., "Longitudinal Associations of Psychosocial Stressors With Menopausal Symptoms and Well-Being Among Women in Midlife," *Menopause* 29, no. 11 (November 2022): 1247–53, doi.org/10.1097/GME.0000000000002056.

54 Beverley Ayers, Mark Forshaw, and Myra S. Hunter, "The Impact of Attitudes Towards the Menopause on Women's Symptom Experience: A Systematic Review," *Maturitas* 65, no. 1 (January 2010): 28–36, doi.org/10.1016/j.maturitas.2009.10.016.

55 Ann Douglas, *Navigating the Messy Middle: A Fiercely Honest and Wildly Encouraging Guide for Midlife Women* (Vancouver: Douglas & McIntyre, 2022), 40–43.

56 Douglas, *Navigating the Messy Middle*, 46.

57 Mosconi et al., "Menopause Impacts Human Brain Structure."

58 Mosconi et al., "Menopause Impacts Human Brain Structure."

59 Gunter, *The Menopause Manifesto*, 150.

60 Nakazawa, *Girls on the Brink*, xiii.

4: What's Truly Broken? How Mental Health Care Has Failed Women

1 Phyllis Chesler, *Women and Madness: Revised and Updated* (New York: St. Martin's Griffin, 2005), 86.

2 Ozlem Eylem et al., "Stigma for Common Mental Disorders in Racial Minorities and Majorities: A Systematic Review and Meta-Analysis," *BMC Public Health* 20 (June 2020): 879, doi.org/10.1186/s12889-020-08964-3.

3 Canadian Institute for Health Information, "1 in 10 Canadians Wait 4 Months or More Before Receiving Community Mental Health Counselling," May 26, 2021, cihi.ca/en/1-in-10-canadians-wait-4-months-or-more-before-receiving-community-mental-health-counselling.

4 Canadian Mental Health Association, "Wait Times for Youth Mental Health Services in Ontario at All-Time High," Canadian Mental Health Association: Ontario, January 27, 2020, ontario.cmha.ca/news/wait-times-for-youth-mental-health-services-in-ontario-at-all-time-high.

5 April Dembosky, "More States Aim to Curb Long Wait Times for Mental Health Care," Benefits Pro, November 29, 2021, benefitspro.com/2021/11/29/more-states-aim-to-curb-long-wait-times-for-mental-health-care.

6 Christina Caron, "'Nobody Has Openings': Mental Health Providers Struggle to Meet Demand," *New York Times*, February 17, 2021, nytimes.com/2021/02/17/well/mind/therapy-appointments-shortages-pandemic.html.

7 Royal College of Psychiatrists, "Two-Fifths of Patients Waiting for Mental Health Treatment Forced to Resort to Emergency or Crisis Services," press

release, October 6, 2020, www.rcpsych.ac.uk/news-and-features/latest-news/detail/2020/10/06/two-fifths-of-patients-waiting-for-mental-health-treatment-forced-to-resort-to-emergency-or-crisis-services.

8   OECD Health Policy Studies, *Waiting Times for Health Services: Next in Line* (Paris: Organisation for Economic Co-operation and Development, 2020), oecd-ilibrary.org/social-issues-migration-health/waiting-times-for-health-services_242e3c8c-en.

9   Statistics Canada, "Mental Health Care Needs, 2018," October 7, 2019, www150.statcan.gc.ca/n1/pub/82-625-x/2019001/article/00011-eng.htm.

10   Jessica Conroy, Luona Lin, and Amrita Ghaness, "Why People Aren't Getting the Care They Need," *Monitor on Psychology* 51, no. 5 (July 2020): 21, apa.org/monitor/2020/07/datapoint-care.

11   Statistics Canada, "Mental Health Care Needs, 2018."

12   Tiffany Lam, "How This Model Reimagines Mental-Health Care for Youth," June 28, 2023, in *In Our Heads*, produced by TVO Today, podcast, 37:24, tvo.org/article/how-this-model-reimagines-mental-health-care-for-youth.

13   David Goldbloom, *We Can Do Better: Urgent Innovations to Improve Mental Health Access and Care* (New York: Simon and Schuster, 2021), 47.

14   Goldbloom, *We Can Do Better*, 47.

15   Michael Mensah, Lucy Ogbu-Nwobodo, and Ruth S. Shim, "Racism and Mental Health Equity: History Repeating Itself," *Psychiatric Services* 72, no. 9 (September 2021): 1091–94, doi.org/10.1176/appi.ps.202000755.

16   Tara F. Bishop, Matthew J. Press, Salomeh Keyhani, and Harold A. Pincus, "Acceptance of Insurance by Psychiatrists and the Implications for Access to Mental Health Care," *JAMA Psychiatry* 71, no. 2 (February 2014): 176–81, doi.org/10.1001/jamapsychiatry.2013.2862.

17   Steve Melek, Stoddard Davenport, and T. J. Gray, *Addiction and Mental Health vs. Physical Health: Widening Disparities in Network Use and Provider Reimbursement* (Milliman, 2019), assets.milliman.com/ektron/Addiction_and_mental_health_vs_physical_health_Widening_disparities_in_network_use_and_provider_reimbursement.pdf.

18   Centers for Medicare and Medicaid Services, "The Mental Health Parity and Addiction Equity Act (MHPAEA)," accessed October 16, 2022, cms.gov/CCIIO/Programs-and-Initiatives/Other-Insurance-Protections/mhpaea_factsheet.

19   U.S. Department of Health and Human Services, "Health Workforce Shortage Areas," 2022, data.hrsa.gov/topics/health-workforce/shortage-areas.

20   Amanda Seitz, "Biden Administration Seeks to Expand 24/7 Mental Health Care," *Toronto Star*, October 18, 2022, thestar.com/news/world/us/2022/10/18/biden-administration-seeks-to-expand-247-mental-health-care.html.

21   The Editorial Board, "The Solution to America's Mental Health Crisis Already Exists," *New York Times*, October 4, 2022, nytimes.com/2022/10/04/opinion/us-mental-health-community-centers.html.

22 Nicholas Moroz, Isabella Moroz, and Monika Slovinec D'Angelo, "Mental Health Services in Canada: Barriers and Cost-Effective Solutions to Increase Access," *Healthcare Management Forum* 33, no. 6 (November 2020): 282–87, doi.org/10.1177/0840470420933911.

23 Denis Campbell and Anna Bawden, "NHS Paying £2bn a Year to Private Hospitals for Mental Health Patients," *The Guardian*, April 24, 2022, theguardian.com/society/2022/apr/24/nhs-paying-2bn-pounds-a-year-to-private-hospitals-for-mental-health-patients.

24 Pamela Jo Johnson, Judy Jou, and Dawn M. Upchurch, "Health Care Disparities Among U.S. Women of Reproductive Age by Level of Psychological Distress," *Journal of Women's Health* 28, no. 9 (September 2019): 1286–94, doi.org/10.1089/jwh.2018.7551.

25 Paula A. Rochon, Nathan M. Stall, and Jerry H. Gurwitz, "Making Older Women Visible," *The Lancet* 397, no. 10268 (January 2021): 21, doi.org/10.1016/S0140-6736(20)32548-4.

26 World Health Organization, "Decade of Healthy Ageing 2020–2030. ZERO Draft," June 12, 2019, who.int/docs/default-source/documents/decade-of-health-ageing/decade-ageing-proposal-en.pdf; Brian W. Ward and Jeannine S. Schiller, "Prevalence of Multiple Chronic Conditions Among US Adults: Estimates From the National Health Interview Survey, 2010," *Preventing Chronic Disease* 10 (April 2013): 120203, doi.org/10.5888/pcd10.120203.

27 Lena D. Sialino et al., "Sex Differences in Mental Health Among Older Adults: Investigating Time Trends and Possible Risk Groups With Regard to Age, Educational Level, and Ethnicity," *Aging & Mental Health* 25, no. 12 (December 2021): 2355–64, doi.org/10.1080/13607863.2020.1847248.

28 Sarah L. Szanton et al., "Effect of Financial Strain on Mortality in Community-Dwelling Older Women," *Journals of Gerontology: Series B* 63, no. 6 (November 2008): S369–74, doi.org/10.1093/geronb/63.6.S369; Ellen Freiberger, Cornel Christian Sieber, and Robert Kob, "Mobility in Older Community-Dwelling Persons: A Narrative Review," *Frontiers in Physiology* 11 (September 2020), doi.org/10.3389/fphys.2020.00881; Annette L. Fitzpatrick et al., "Barriers to Health Care Access Among the Elderly and Who Perceives Them," *American Journal of Public Health* 94, no. 10 (October 2004): 1788–94, doi.org/10.2105/ajph.94.10.1788.

29 Behzad Karami Matin et al., "Barriers in Access to Healthcare for Women With Disabilities: A Systematic Review in Qualitative Studies," *BMC Women's Health* 21 (January 2021): 44, doi.org/10.1186/s12905-021-01189-5; Hilary K. Brown et al., "Disability and Interpersonal Violence in the Perinatal Period," *Obstetrics & Gynecology* 140, no. 5 (November 2022): 797–805, doi.org/10.1097/AOG.0000000000004950.

30 Robin Bleiweis, Diana Boesch, and Alexandra Cawthorne Gaines, "The Basic Facts About Women in Poverty," Center for American Progress, August 3, 2020, americanprogress.org/article/basic-facts-women-poverty.

31 Statistics Canada, "Percentage of Persons in Low Income by Sex," Table 11-10-0135-02, May 2, 2023, www150.statcan.gc.ca/t1/tbl1/en/ tv.action?pid=1110013502.

32 American Psychiatric Association, "Mental Health Disparities: Diverse Populations," accessed December 1, 2021, psychiatry.org/psychiatrists/ diversity/education/mental-health-facts.

33 American Psychological Association, "Ethnic and Racial Minorities and Socioeconomic Status," 2017, apa.org/pi/ses/resources/publications/minorities.

34 Rhea Wyse et al., "Diversity by Race, Ethnicity, and Sex Within the US Psychiatry Physician Workforce," *Academic Psychiatry* 44, no. 5 (October 2020): 523–30, doi.org/10.1007/s40596-020-01276-z.

35 Henna Budhwani, Kristine Ria Hearld, and Daniel Chavez-Yenter, "Depression in Racial and Ethnic Minorities: The Impact of Nativity and Discrimination," *Journal of Racial and Ethnic Health Disparities* 2, no. 1 (March 2015): 34–42, doi.org/10.1007/s40615-014-0045-z.

36 Erik J. Rodriquez et al., "Relationships Between Allostatic Load, Unhealthy Behaviors, and Depressive Disorder in U.S. Adults, 2005–2012 NHANES," *Preventive Medicine* 110 (May 2018): 9–15, doi.org/10.1016/j.ypmed.2018.02.002.

37 Zohaib Sohail, Rahn Kennedy Bailey, and William D. Richie, "Misconceptions of Depression in African Americans," *Frontiers in Psychiatry* 5 (June 2014), doi.org/10.3389/fpsyt.2014.00065; Rahn Kennedy Bailey, Josephine Mokonogho, and Alok Kumar, "Racial and Ethnic Differences in Depression: Current Perspectives," *Neuropsychiatric Disease and Treatment* 15 (February 2019): 603–9, doi.org/10.2147/NDT.S128584.

38 American Psychiatric Association, "Mental Health Disparities."

39 Eylem et al., "Stigma for Common Mental Disorders."

40 Erum Nadeem et al., "Does Stigma Keep Poor Young Immigrant and U.S.-Born Black and Latina Women From Seeking Mental Health Care?," *Psychiatric Services* 58, no. 12 (December 2007): 1547–54, doi.org/10.1176/ps.2007.58.12.1547.

41 Lindsay Wong, *The Woo-Woo: How I Survived Ice Hockey, Drug Raids, Demons, and My Crazy Chinese Family* (Vancouver: Arsenal Pulp Press, 2018).

42 Leonor Ward et al., "A Process of Healing for the Labrador Innu: Improving Health and Wellbeing in the Context of Historical and Contemporary Colonialism," *Social Science & Medicine* 279 (June 2021): 113973, doi.org/ 10.1016/j.socscimed.2021.113973.

43 Resmaa Menakem, *My Grandmother's Hands: Racialized Trauma and the Pathway to Mending Our Hearts and Bodies* (Las Vegas: Central Recovery Press, 2017), xviii–xix.

44 Resmaa Menakem, "White Supremacy as a Trauma Response," Medium (blog), April 14, 2018, medium.com/@rmenakem/white-supremacy-as-a-trauma-response-ce631b82b975.

45 Elinor Cleghorn, *Unwell Women: Misdiagnosis and Myth in a Man-Made World* (New York: Dutton, 2021), 266.

46 Kelly M. Hoffman, Sophie Trawalter, Jordan R. Axt, and M. Norman Oliver, "Racial Bias in Pain Assessment and Treatment Recommendations, and False Beliefs About Biological Differences Between Blacks and Whites," *Proceedings of the National Academy of Sciences* 113, no. 16 (April 19, 2016): 4296–301, doi.org/10.1073/pnas.1516047113.

47 Menakem, *My Grandmother's Hands*, 108.

48 Janette Dill and Mignon Duffy, "Structural Racism and Black Women's Employment in the US Health Care Sector," *Health Affairs* 41, no. 2 (February 2022): 265–72, doi.org/10.1377/hlthaff.2021.01400.

49 Luona Lin, Karen Stamm, and Peggy Christidis, "How Diverse Is the Psychology Workforce?," *Monitor on Psychology* 49, no. 2 (February 2018): 19, apa.org/monitor/2018/02/datapoint.

50 Dill and Duffy, "Structural Racism."

51 Stephanie Castelin and Grace White, "'I'm a Strong Independent Black Woman': The Strong Black Woman Schema and Mental Health in College-Aged Black Women," *Psychology of Women Quarterly* 46, no. 2 (June 2022): 196–208, doi.org/10.1177/03616843211067501.

52 Marita Golden, *The Strong Black Woman: How a Myth Endangers the Physical and Mental Health of Black Women* (Coral Gables, FL: Mango, 2021), 65.

53 Hermioni N. Lokko, Justin A. Chen, Ranna I. Parekh, and Theodore A. Stern, "Racial and Ethnic Diversity in the US Psychiatric Workforce: A Perspective and Recommendations," *Academic Psychiatry* 40, no. 6 (December 2016): 898–904, doi.org/10.1007/s40596-016-0591-2.

54 Krystal Kavita Jagoo, "What Does Anti-Oppressive Therapy Look Like?," *Asparagus Magazine*, June 16, 2021, asparagusmagazine.com/articles/toronto-wellnest-mental-health-clinic-offers-anti-oppressive-counselling-for-racialized-communities.

55 Yesenia Merino, Leslie Adams, and William J. Hall, "Implicit Bias and Mental Health Professionals: Priorities and Directions for Research," *Psychiatric Services* 69, no. 6 (June 2018): 723–25, doi.org/10.1176/appi.ps.201700294.

56 John B. McKinlay, "A Case for Refocusing Upstream: The Political Economy of Illness," in *The Sociology of Health and Illness: Critical Perspectives*, 7th ed. (New York: Worth Publishers, 2005), 551–64, iaphs.org/wp-content/uploads/2019/11/IAPHS-McKinlay-Article.pdf.

57 Faraaz Mahomed, "Addressing the Problem of Severe Underinvestment in Mental Health and Well-Being From a Human Rights Perspective," *Health and Human Rights* 22, no. 1 (June 2020): 35–49, ncbi.nlm.nih.gov/pmc/articles/PMC7348439.

58 Mahomed, "Addressing the Problem of Severe Underinvestment."

59 Shridhar Sharma, "Psychiatry, Colonialism and Indian Civilization: A Historical Appraisal," *Indian Journal of Psychiatry* 48, no. 2 (April–June 2006): 109–12, doi.org/10.4103/0019-5545.31600.

60 "Origin Story: Who Is 'Bapu'?," Bapu Trust for Research on Mind and Discourse, 2020, baputrust.com/origin-story.

61   Bhargavi V. Davar, Kavita Pillai, and Kimberly LaCroix, "Seher's 'Circle of Care'
      Model in Advancing Supported Decision Making in India," in *Mental Health,
      Legal Capacity, and Human Rights*, ed. Michael Ashley Stein et al. (Cambridge, UK:
      Cambridge University Press, 2021), 213–29, doi.org/10.1017/9781108979016.017.

62   Davar, Pillai, and LaCroix, "Seher's 'Circle of Care.'"

63   WHO Western Pacific, "A Toolkit on How to Implement Social Prescribing,"
      World Health Organization Western Pacific, May 20, 2022, who.int/
      publications/i/item/9789290619765.

64   Henry Aughterson, Louise Baxter, and Daisy Fancourt, "Social Prescribing
      for Individuals With Mental Health Problems: A Qualitative Study of Barriers
      and Enablers Experienced by General Practitioners," *BMC Family Practice* 21
      (September 2020): 194, doi.org/10.1186/s12875-020-01264-0.

5: The Cultural Construction of Mental Illness

1   Yaa Gyasi, *Transcendent Kingdom* (New York: Knopf, 2020), 37.

2   Giovanni A. Fava and Nicoletta Sonino, "The Biopsychosocial Model Thirty
     Years Later," *Psychotherapy and Psychosomatics* 77, no. 1 (December 2007): 1–2,
     doi.org/10.1159/000110052.

3   Allan H. Ropper and Brian David Burrell, *How the Brain Lost Its Mind: Sex,
     Hysteria, and the Riddle of Mental Illness* (New York: Avery, 2019), 211.

4   Ropper and Burrell, *How the Brain Lost Its Mind*, 8.

5   Joshua J. Kemp, James J. Lickel, and Brett J. Deacon, "Effects of a Chemical
     Imbalance Causal Explanation on Individuals' Perceptions of Their
     Depressive Symptoms," *Behaviour Research and Therapy* 56 (May 2014): 47–52,
     doi.org/10.1016/j.brat.2014.02.009.

6   Hans S. Schroder et al., "Stressors and Chemical Imbalances: Beliefs About
     the Causes of Depression in an Acute Psychiatric Treatment Sample," *Journal
     of Affective Disorders* 276 (November 2020): 537–45, doi.org/10.1016/j.
     jad.2020.07.061.

7   Jussi Valtonen, Woo-kyoung Ahn, and Andrei Cimpian, "Neurodualism:
     People Assume That the Brain Affects the Mind More Than the Mind
     Affects the Brain," *Cognitive Science* 45, no. 9 (September 2021): e13034,
     doi.org/10.1111/cogs.13034.

8   Ropper and Burrell, *How the Brain Lost Its Mind*, 199.

9   Ropper and Burrell, *How the Brain Lost Its Mind*, 194–95.

10   Kristen L. Syme and Edward H. Hagen, "Mental Health Is Biological
      Health: Why Tackling 'Diseases of the Mind' Is an Imperative for Biological
      Anthropology in the 21st Century," *American Journal of Biological Anthropology*
      171, no. S70 (May 2020): 87–117, doi.org/10.1002/ajpa.23965.

11   Joseph J. McCann, "Is Mental Illness Socially Constructed?," *Journal of Applied
      Psychology and Social Science* 2, no. 1 (2016): 1–11, insight.cumbria.ac.uk/id/
      eprint/2203/1/McCann_IsMentalIllness.pdf.

12 Syme and Hagen, "Mental Health Is Biological Health"; Ropper and Burrell, *How the Brain Lost Its Mind*, 26.

13 Alex Riley, *A Cure for Darkness: The Story of Depression and How We Treat It* (New York: Scribner, 2021), 42.

14 Riley, *A Cure for Darkness*, 83.

15 Canadian Mental Health Association, "*DSM-5* Released Amidst Controversy," CMHA, May 30, 2013, ontario.cmha.ca/news/dsm-5-released-amidst-controversy.

16 Jonathan Foiles, *(Mis)Diagnosed: How Bias Distorts Our Perception of Mental Health* (Cleveland: Belt Publishing, 2021), 18.

17 Foiles, *(Mis)Diagnosed*, 18.

18 Foiles, *(Mis)Diagnosed*, 93–94.

19 Yale School of Medicine, "A Theory Abandoned but Still Compelling," *Yale Medicine Magazine*, Autumn 2008, medicine.yale.edu/news/yale-medicine-magazine/article/a-theory-abandoned-but-still-compelling.

20 Ropper and Burrell, *How the Brain Lost Its Mind*, 107.

21 Jonathan Foiles, "Gender, Stigma, and Bias: Everything We Get Wrong About Borderline Personality Disorder," *Literary Hub*, September 9, 2021, lithub.com/gender-stigma-and-bias-everything-we-get-wrong-about-borderline-personality-disorder.

22 Foiles, "Gender, Stigma, and Bias."

23 Andrew E. Skodol and Donna S. Bender, "Why Are Women Diagnosed Borderline More Than Men?," *Psychiatric Quarterly* 74, no. 4 (December 2003): 349–60, doi.org/10.1023/a:1026087410516.

24 Bridget F. Grant et al., "Prevalence, Correlates, Disability, and Comorbidity of *DSM-IV* Borderline Personality Disorder: Results From the Wave 2 National Epidemiologic Survey on Alcohol and Related Conditions," *Journal of Clinical Psychiatry* 69, no. 4 (April 2008): 533–45, doi.org/10.4088/jcp.v69n0404.

25 Craig Rodriguez-Seijas, Theresa A. Morgan, and Mark Zimmerman, "Is There a Bias in the Diagnosis of Borderline Personality Disorder Among Lesbian, Gay, and Bisexual Patients?," *Assessment* 28, no. 3 (April 2021): 724–38, doi.org/10.1177/1073191120961833.

26 Jayashri Kulkarni and Patrick Walker, "We Need to Treat Borderline Personality Disorder for What It Really Is—a Response to Trauma," *The Conversation*, May 2, 2019, theconversation.com/we-need-to-treat-borderline-personality-disorder-for-what-it-really-is-a-response-to-trauma-115549.

27 Robert B. Dudas et al., "The Overlap Between Autistic Spectrum Conditions and Borderline Personality Disorder," *PLOS ONE* 12, no. 9 (September 2017): e0184447, doi.org/10.1371/journal.pone.0184447.

28 Denny Borsboom and Angélique O. J. Cramer, "Network Analysis: An Integrative Approach to the Structure of Psychopathology," *Annual Review of Clinical Psychology* 9 (2013): 91–121, doi.org/10.1146/annurev-clinpsy-050212-185608. The network map of mental disorders is available under "Supplemental Material."

29 Denny Borsboom, "A Network Theory of Mental Disorders," *World Psychiatry* 16, no. 1 (February 2017): 5–13, doi.org/10.1002/wps.20375.

30 Mental Health Commission of Canada, "Workplace Mental Health," Mental Health Commission of Canada, accessed November 9, 2021, mentalhealthcommission.ca/what-we-do/workplace.

31 Erica Alini, "'I Couldn't Believe It'—Why Disability Claims for Mental Health Are Often a Struggle," Global News, May 25, 2019, globalnews.ca/news/5306210/disability-insurance-mental-health.

32 Joanna Moncrieff et al., "The Serotonin Theory of Depression: A Systematic Umbrella Review of the Evidence," *Molecular Psychiatry* (July 20, 2022), doi.org/10.1038/s41380-022-01661-0.

33 Ana Sabela Álvarez, Marco Pagani, and Paolo Meucci, "The Clinical Application of the Biopsychosocial Model in Mental Health: A Research Critique," *American Journal of Physical Medicine & Rehabilitation* 91, no. 13 (February 2012): S173–80, doi.org/10.1097/PHM.0b013e31823d54be.

34 George L. Engel, "The Need for a New Medical Model: A Challenge for Biomedicine," *Science* 196, no. 4286 (April 8, 1977): 129–36, doi.org/10.1126/science.847460.

35 Fava and Sonino, "The Biopsychosocial Model Thirty Years Later."

36 Sanah Ahsan, "I'm a Psychologist—and I Believe We've Been Told Devastating Lies About Mental Health," *The Guardian*, September 6, 2022, theguardian.com/commentisfree/2022/sep/06/psychologist-devastating-lies-mental-health-problems-politics.

6: The Problems With Patriarchy

1 Audre Lorde, "The Uses of Anger: Women Responding to Racism," republished on BlackPast.org, August 12, 2012, blackpast.org/african-american-history/speeches-african-american-history/1981-audre-lorde-uses-anger-women-responding-racism.

2 Holly Corbett, "#MeToo Five Years Later: How the Movement Started and What Needs to Change," *Forbes*, October 27, 2022, forbes.com/sites/hollycorbett/2022/10/27/metoo-five-years-later-how-the-movement-started-and-what-needs-to-change.

3 Zenobia Jeffries Warfield, "Me Too Creator Tarana Burke Reminds Us This Is About Black and Brown Survivors," *Yes!*, January 4, 2018, yesmagazine.org/democracy/2018/01/04/me-too-creator-tarana-burke-reminds-us-this-is-about-black-and-brown-survivors.

4 Statistics Canada, "Gender-Based Violence and Unwanted Sexual Behaviour in Canada, 2018: Initial Findings From the Survey of Safety in Public and Private Spaces," December 5, 2019, www150.statcan.gc.ca/n1/daily-quotidien/191205/dq191205b-eng.htm.

5   World Health Organization, "Devastatingly Pervasive: 1 in 3 Women Globally
    Experience Violence," news release, March 9, 2021, who.int/news/item/09-03-
    2021-devastatingly-pervasive-1-in-3-women-globally-experience-violence.

6   Davey M. Smith, Nicole E. Johns, and Anita Raj, "Do Sexual Minorities Face
    Greater Risk for Sexual Harassment, Ever and at School in Adolescence?
    Findings From a 2019 Cross-Sectional Study of U.S. Adults," *Journal of
    Interpersonal Violence* 37, no. 3–4 (February 2022): NP1963–87, doi.org/
    10.1177/0886260520926315; Jameta Nicole Barlow, "Black Women,
    the Forgotten Survivors of Sexual Assault," American Psychological
    Association, February 1, 2020, apa.org/pi/about/newsletter/2020/02/
    black-women-sexual-assault.

7   Amnesty International, "Missing and Murdered Indigenous Women and
    Girls: The Facts," January 29, 2021, amnesty.ca/blog/missing-and-murdered-
    indigenous-women-facts; Native Women's Association of Canada, *NWAC
    Action Plan: Our Calls, Our Action*, 2021, nwac.ca/assets-knowledge-centre/
    NWAC-action-plan-English.pdf.

8   Therése Skoog and Sevgi Bayram Özdemir, "Explaining Why Early-Maturing
    Girls Are More Exposed to Sexual Harassment in Early Adolescence," *Journal
    of Early Adolescence* 36, no. 4 (May 2016): 490–509, doi.org/10.1177/
    0272431614568198.

9   Jane Mendle, Rebecca M. Ryan, and Kirsten M. P. McKone, "Age at Menarche,
    Depression, and Antisocial Behavior in Adulthood," *Pediatrics* 141, no. 1
    (January 2018): e20171703, doi.org/10.1542/peds.2017-1703.

10 "Welcome," Everyone's Invited, everyonesinvited.uk.

11 Ofsted, "Review of Sexual Abuse in Schools and Colleges," Government of the
    United Kingdom Office for Standards in Education, Children's Services,
    and Skills, June 10, 2021, gov.uk/government/publications/review-of-sexual-
    abuse-in-schools-and-colleges/review-of-sexual-abuse-in-schools-and-colleges.

12 Dagmar Stockman et al., "An Ecological Approach to Understanding the
    Impact of Sexual Violence: A Systematic Meta-Review," *Frontiers in Psychology*
    14 (2023), doi.org/10.3389/fpsyg.2023.1032408.

13 Miranda Olff, "Sex and Gender Differences in Post-Traumatic Stress Disorder:
    An Update," *European Journal of Psychotraumatology* 8, sup4 (2017): 1351204,
    doi.org/10.1080/20008198.2017.1351204.

14 Donna Jackson Nakazawa, *Girls on the Brink: Helping Our Daughters Thrive in an Era
    of Increased Anxiety, Depression, and Social Media* (New York: Harmony, 2022), 72.

15 George M. Slavich, "Social Safety Theory: A Biologically Based Evolutionary
    Perspective on Life Stress, Health, and Behavior," *Annual Review of Clinical
    Psychology* 16, no. 1 (2020): 265–95, doi.org/10.1146/annurev-clinpsy-032816-045159.

16 Nakazawa, *Girls on the Brink*, 72.

17   Kristen L. Syme and Edward H. Hagen, "Most Anguish Isn't an Illness but an Evolved Response to Adversity," *Psyche*, September 29, 2020, psyche.co/ideas/most-anguish-isnt-an-illness-but-an-evolved-response-to-adversity.

18   Lisa Feldman Barrett, "Your Brain Secretly Works With Other Brains," *Mindful*, September 16, 2021, mindful.org/why-your-breath-is-connected-to-your-well-being-2.

19   Feldman Barrett, "Your Brain Secretly Works."

20   Edward H. Hagen and Kristen L. Syme, "Credible Sadness, Coercive Sadness: Depression as a Functional Response to Adversity and Strife," in *The Oxford Handbook of Evolution and the Emotions*, eds. Laith Al-Shawaf and Todd Shackelford (Oxford, UK: Oxford University Press, 2023).

21   Centers for Disease Control and Prevention, "Fast Facts: Preventing Adverse Childhood Experiences," Centers for Disease Control and Prevention, April 6, 2021, cdc.gov/violenceprevention/aces/fastfact.html.

22   Nakazawa, *Girls on the Brink*, 101.

23   Alexandra Burza, "How Can Personalized Medicine for Psychological Trauma Help Reconnect the Mind and Body?," Western University Schulich Medicine and Dentistry Research Office, accessed December 4, 2022, schulich.uwo.ca/research/research_excellence/daring_to_ask/endowed_chairs/dr_ruth_lanius.html.

24   Julie Lalonde, *Resilience Is Futile: The Life and Death and Life of Julie S. Lalonde* (Toronto: Between the Lines, 2020).

25   Aubrey Gordon, *What We Don't Talk About When We Talk About Fat* (Boston: Beacon Press, 2020), 102.

26   Glennon Doyle, Abby Wambach, and Amanda Doyle, "Ep 156: Jane F-ing Fonda," December 1, 2022, in *We Can Do Hard Things*, produced by Cadence 13, podcast, 52:14, momastery.com/blog/we-can-do-hard-things-ep-156.

27   Thomas Curran and Andrew P. Hill, "Perfectionism Is Increasing Over Time: A Meta-Analysis of Birth Cohort Differences From 1989 to 2016," *Psychological Bulletin* 145, no. 4 (April 2019): 410–29, doi.org/10.1037/bul0000138.

28   Curran and Hill, "Perfectionism Is Increasing."

29   Liv Sand et al., "Perfectionism in Adolescence: Associations With Gender, Age, and Socioeconomic Status in a Norwegian Sample," *Frontiers in Public Health* 9 (2021): 688811, doi.org/10.3389/fpubh.2021.688811.

30   Chang Chen, Paul L. Hewitt, and Gordon L. Flett, "Adverse Childhood Experiences and Multidimensional Perfectionism in Young Adults," *Personality and Individual Differences* 146 (August 2019): 53–57, doi.org/10.1016/j.paid.2019.03.042.

31   Patricia Marten DiBartolo and María José Rendón, "A Critical Examination of the Construct of Perfectionism and Its Relationship to Mental Health in Asian and African Americans Using a Cross-Cultural Framework," *Clinical Psychology Review* 32, no. 3 (April 2012): 139–52, doi.org/10.1016/j.cpr.2011.09.007.

32 Tema Okun, "White Supremacy Culture," Dismantling Racism Works Web
Work, accessed January 14, 2023, whitesupremacyculture.info/uploads/
4/3/5/7/43579015/okun_-_white_sup_culture.pdf.

33 Robert C. Whitaker et al., "The Interaction of Adverse Childhood Experiences
and Gender as Risk Factors for Depression and Anxiety Disorders in US Adults:
A Cross-Sectional Study," *BMC Public Health* 21, no. 1 (December 2021): 2078,
doi.org/10.1186/s12889-021-12058-z.

34 Charlene Y. Senn et al., "Secondary and 2-Year Outcomes of a Sexual Assault
Resistance Program for University Women," *Psychology of Women Quarterly* 41,
no. 2 (June 2017): 147–62, doi.org/10.1177/0361684317690119.

7: Are You Mentally Ill or Mentally Overloaded?

1 Denise Comanne, "How Patriarchy and Capitalism Combine to Aggravate
the Oppression of Women," Committee for the Abolition of Illegitimate Debt,
May 28, 2020, cadtm.org/How-Patriarchy-and-Capitalism-Combine-to-
Aggravate-the-Oppression-of-Women.

2 Gemma Hartley, *Fed Up: Emotional Labor, Women, and the Way Forward* (New
York: HarperOne, 2018), 13.

3 Lyn Craig and Brendan Churchill, "Working and Caring at Home: Gender
Differences in the Effects of COVID-19 on Paid and Unpaid Labor in Australia,"
Feminist Economics 27, no. 1–2 (2021): 310–26, doi.org/10.1080/13545701.2020.1831039.

4 Liz Dean, Brendan Churchill, and Leah Ruppanner, "The Mental Load:
Building a Deeper Theoretical Understanding of How Cognitive and
Emotional Labor Over*load* Women and Mothers," *Community, Work & Family*
25, no. 1 (2022): 13–29, doi.org/10.1080/13668803.2021.2002813.

5 Dean, Churchill, and Ruppanner, "The Mental Load."

6 Eve Rodsky, *Fair Play: A Game-Changing Solution for When You Have Too Much
to Do (and More Life to Live)* (New York: G. P. Putnam's Sons, 2019).

7 Jean Duncombe and Dennis Marsden, "'Workaholics' and 'Whingeing
Women': Theorising Intimacy and Emotion Work—the Last Frontier of
Gender Inequality?," *Sociological Review* 43, no. 1 (February 1995): 150–69,
doi.org/10.1111/j.1467-954X.1995.tb02482.x.

8 Francesca Donner, "The Household Work Men and Women Do, and Why,"
New York Times, February 12, 2020, nytimes.com/2020/02/12/us/the-
household-work-men-and-women-do-and-why.html.

9 Duncombe and Marsden, "'Workaholics' and 'Whingeing Women.'"

10 Melanie E. Brewster, "Lesbian Women and Household Labor Division: A
Systematic Review of Scholarly Research From 2000 to 2015," *Journal of Lesbian
Studies* 21, no. 1 (January 2017): 47–69, doi.org/10.1080/10894160.2016.1142350.

11 Claire Cain Miller, "How Same-Sex Couples Divide Chores, and What It Reveals
About Modern Parenting," *New York Times*, May 16, 2018, nytimes.com/
2018/05/16/upshot/same-sex-couples-divide-chores-much-more-evenly-until-
they-become-parents.html.

12 Brigid Schulte, *Overwhelmed: How to Work, Love, and Play When No One Has the Time* (New York: Macmillan Publishers, 2014), 73.

13 Amanda Wilkinson, "So Wives Didn't Work in the 'Good Old Days'? Wrong," *The Guardian*, April 13, 2014, theguardian.com/commentisfree/2014/apr/13/working-women-stay-at-home-wives-myths.

14 Schulte, *Overwhelmed*, 76–77.

15 Catherine Verniers, Virginie Bonnot, and Yvette Assilaméhou-Kunz, "Intensive Mothering and the Perpetuation of Gender Inequality: Evidence From a Mixed Methods Research," *Acta Psychologica* 227 (July 2022) : 103614, doi.org/10.1016/j.actpsy.2022.103614.

16 Verniers, Bonnot, and Assilaméhou-Kunz, "Intensive Mothering."

17 World Health Organization, "Burn-Out an 'Occupational Phenomenon': International Classification of Diseases," May 28, 2019, who.int/news/item/28-05-2019-burn-out-an-occupational-phenomenon-international-classification-of-diseases.

18 Nancy Beauregard et al., "Gendered Pathways to Burnout: Results From the SALVEO Study," *Annals of Work Exposures and Health* 62, no. 4 (May 2018): 426–37, doi.org/10.1093/annweh/wxx114.

19 Kate Morgan, "Why In-Person Workers May Be More Likely to Get Promoted," BBC News, March 7, 2021, bbc.com/worklife/article/20210305-why-in-person-workers-may-be-more-likely-to-get-promoted.

20 Allyson Chiu, "How to Know If You're a People-Pleaser and What to Do About It," *Washington Post*, September 8, 2022, washingtonpost.com/wellness/2022/06/15/people-pleaser-personality-psychology.

21 Linda Babcock et al., *The No Club: Putting a Stop to Women's Dead-End Work* (New York: Simon & Schuster, 2022), 58–65.

22 Panagiota Koutsimani, Anthony Montgomery, and Katerina Georganta, "The Relationship Between Burnout, Depression, and Anxiety: A Systematic Review and Meta-Analysis," *Frontiers in Psychology* 10 (2019): 284, doi.org/10.3389/fpsyg.2019.00284; Irvin Sam Schonfeld and Renzo Bianchi, "Burnout and Depression: Two Entities or One?," *Journal of Clinical Psychology* 72, no. 1 (January 2016): 22–37, doi.org/10.1002/jclp.22229.

23 Andrea M. Stelnicki et al., "Associations Between Burnout and Mental Disorder Symptoms Among Nurses in Canada," *Canadian Journal of Nursing Research* 53, no. 3 (September 2021): 254–63, doi.org/10.1177/0844562120974194.

24 Taina Hintsa et al., "Is There an Independent Association Between Burnout and Increased Allostatic Load? Testing the Contribution of Psychological Distress and Depression," *Journal of Health Psychology* 21, no. 8 (August 2016): 1576–86, doi.org/10.1177/1359105314559619.

25 Koutsimani, Montgomery, and Georganta, "The Relationship Between Burnout, Depression, and Anxiety."

26 Aisha Harris, "A History of Self-Care," *Slate*, April 5, 2017, slate.com/articles/arts/culturebox/2017/04/the_history_of_self_care.html.

27 Kathryn Dean, "Self-Care Components of Lifestyles: The Importance of Gender, Attitudes and the Social Situation," *Social Science & Medicine* 29, no. 2 (1989): 137–52, doi.org/10.1016/0277-9536(89)90162-7.

28 Carlyn M. Hood, Keith P. Gennuso, Geoffrey R. Swain, and Bridget B. Catlin, "County Health Rankings: Relationships Between Determinant Factors and Health Outcomes," *American Journal of Preventive Medicine* 50, no. 2 (February 2016): 129–35, doi.org/10.1016/j.amepre.2015.08.024.

29 J. L. Kuk et al., "Individuals With Obesity but No Other Metabolic Risk Factors Are Not at Significantly Elevated All-Cause Mortality Risk in Men and Women," *Clinical Obesity* 8 no. 5 (October 2018): 305–12, doi.org/10.1111/cob.12263.

30 Long Ge et al., "Comparison of Dietary Macronutrient Patterns of 14 Popular Named Dietary Programmes for Weight and Cardiovascular Risk Factor Reduction in Adults: Systematic Review and Network Meta-Analysis of Randomised Trials," *BMJ* 369, no. 8240 (April 4, 2020): m696, doi.org/10.1136/bmj.m696.

31 Aisha Harris, "A History of Self-Care."

32 Sarah Riley, Adrienne Evans, Emma Anderson, and Martine Robson, "The Gendered Nature of Self-Help," *Feminism & Psychology* 29, no. 1 (February 2019): 3–18, doi.org/10.1177/0959353519826162.

33 Riley et al., "The Gendered Nature of Self-Help."

34 Bethany L. Johnson and Margaret M. Quinlan, *You're Doing It Wrong! Mothering, Media, and Medical Expertise* (New Brunswick, NJ: Rutgers University Press, 2019), 43.

35 Yael Chatav Schonbrun, "A Mother's Ambitions," Opinionator, *New York Times*, July 30, 2014, opinionator.blogs.nytimes.com/2014/07/30/a-mothers-ambitions.

36 William M. Kenkel, Allison M. Perkeybile, and C. Sue Carter, "The Neurobiological Causes and Effects of Alloparenting," *Developmental Neurobiology* 77, no. 2 (February 2017): 214–32, doi.org/10.1002/dneu.22465.

37 Yael Schonbrun and Rebecca Schrag Hershberg, "The Pandemic Should Encourage a New Alloparenting Future," *Behavioral Scientist*, May 17, 2021, behavioralscientist.org/the-pandemic-should-encourage-a-new-alloparenting-future.

38 Dean, Churchill, and Ruppanner, "The Mental Load."

39 Tricia Hersey, *Rest Is Resistance: A Manifesto* (New York: Little, Brown Spark, 2022).

40 Matthew Desmond, "American Capitalism Is Brutal. You Can Trace That to the Plantation," *New York Times*, August 14, 2019, nytimes.com/interactive/2019/08/14/magazine/slavery-capitalism.html.

41 Hersey, *Rest Is Resistance*, 23.

42 Saundra Dalton-Smith, "The Real Reason Why We Are Tired and What to Do About It," filmed in Atlanta, GA, TEDx video, 2019, 9:34, youtube.com/watch?v=ZGNN4EPJzGk.

43 Marissa Goldberg, "Rest Isn't the Opposite of Work," *Remote Work Prep* (blog), accessed January 15, 2023, remoteworkprep.com/blog/rest-isnt-the-opposite-of-work.

8: The Promises (and Pitfalls) of Therapy

1   Josef Breuer and Sigmund Freud, *Studies on Hysteria* (New York: Basic Book Publishers, 1891): 305, archive.org/details/studiesonhysteri037649mbp/page/n341/mode/2up.

2   Alex Riley, *A Cure for Darkness: The Story of Depression and How We Treat It* (New York: Scribner, 2021), 210–212.

3   Stefan G. Hofmann et al., "The Efficacy of Cognitive Behavioral Therapy: A Review of Meta-Analyses," *Cognitive Therapy and Research* 36, no. 5 (October 2012): 427–40, doi.org/10.1007/s10608-012-9476-1.

4   Liliane Cambraia Windsor, Alexis Jemal, and Edward Alessi, "Cognitive Behavioral Therapy: A Meta-Analysis of Race and Substance Use Outcomes," *Cultural Diversity & Ethnic Minority Psychology* 21, no. 2 (April 2015): 300–13, doi.org/10.1037/a0037929.

5   Windsor, Jemal, and Alessi, "Cognitive Behavioral Therapy."

6   Leif Tore Moberg, Birgitte Solvang, Rannveig Grøm Sæle, and Anna Dahl Myrvang, "Effects of Cognitive-Behavioral and Psychodynamic-Interpersonal Treatments for Eating Disorders: A Meta-Analytic Inquiry into the Role of Patient Characteristics and Change in Eating Disorder-Specific and General Psychopathology in Remission," *Journal of Eating Disorders* 9, no. 1 (2021): 74, doi.org/10.1186/s40337-021-00430-8.

7   Leman Kaniturk Kose, Lise Fox, and Eric A. Storch, "Effectiveness of Cognitive Behavioral Therapy for Individuals With Autism Spectrum Disorders and Comorbid Obsessive-Compulsive Disorder: A Review of the Research," *Journal of Developmental and Physical Disabilities* 30, no. 1 (February 2018): 69–87, doi.org/10.1007/s10882-017-9559-8.

8   Mariya V. Cherkasova et al., "Efficacy of Cognitive Behavioral Therapy With and Without Medication for Adults With ADHD: A Randomized Clinical Trial," *Journal of Attention Disorders* 24, no. 6 (April 2020): 889–903, doi.org/10.1177/1087054716671197.

9   Ruth von Brachel et al., "Long-Term Effectiveness of Cognitive Behavioral Therapy in Routine Outpatient Care: A 5- to 20-Year Follow-Up Study," *Psychotherapy and Psychosomatics* 88, no. 4 (August 2019): 222–35, doi.org/10.1159/000500188.

10 Bessel van der Kolk, *The Body Keeps the Score: Brain, Mind, and Body in the Healing of Trauma* (New York: Penguin Books, 2015); Resmaa Menakem, *My Grandmother's Hands: Racialized Trauma and the Pathway to Mending Our Hearts and Bodies* (Las Vegas: Central Recovery Press, 2017); Minke M. van de Kamp et al., "Body- and Movement-Oriented Interventions for Posttraumatic Stress Disorder: A Systematic Review and Meta Analysis," *Journal of Traumatic Stress* 32, no. 6 (December 2019): 967–76, doi.org/10.1002/jts.22465.

11 Richard P. Dum, David J. Levinthal, and Peter L. Strick, "Motor, Cognitive, and Affective Areas of the Cerebral Cortex Influence the Adrenal Medulla,"

Proceedings of the National Academy of Sciences 113, no. 35 (August 30, 2016): 9922–27, doi.org/10.1073/pnas.1605044113.

12 "New Insights Into How the Mind Influences the Body," *ScienceDaily*, August 15, 2016, sciencedaily.com/releases/2016/08/160815185555.htm.

13 Menakem, *My Grandmother's Hands*, 13.

14 Hillary L. McBride, *The Wisdom of Your Body: Finding Healing, Wholeness and Connection Through Embodied Living* (Toronto: Collins, 2021), 67.

15 Bahareh Eslami et al., "Lifetime Abuse and Somatic Symptoms Among Older Women and Men in Europe," *PLOS ONE* 14, no. 8 (August 8, 2019): e0220741, doi.org/10.1371/journal.pone.0220741.

16 Marylène Cloitre, "ICD-11 Complex Post-Traumatic Stress Disorder: Simplifying Diagnosis in Trauma Populations," *British Journal of Psychiatry* 216, no. 3 (March 2020): 129–31, doi.org/10.1192/bjp.2020.43.

17 APA, "What Is Exposure Therapy?," American Psychological Association, accessed February 11, 2022, apa.org/ptsd-guideline/patients-and-families/exposure-therapy.

18 Marie Kuhfuß et al., "Somatic Experiencing—Effectiveness and Key Factors of a Body-Oriented Trauma Therapy: A Scoping Literature Review," *European Journal of Psychotraumatology* 12, no. 1 (January 1, 2021): 1929023, doi.org/10.1080/20008198.2021.1929023.

19 Cynthia J. Price and Helen Y. Weng, "Facilitating Adaptive Emotion Processing and Somatic Reappraisal via Sustained Mindful Interoceptive Attention," *Frontiers in Psychology* 12 (2021): 578827, doi.org/10.3389/fpsyg.2021.578827.

20 Cynthia J. Price and Carole Hooven, "Interoceptive Awareness Skills for Emotion Regulation: Theory and Approach of Mindful Awareness in Body-Oriented Therapy (MABT)," *Frontiers in Psychology* 9 (2018): 798, doi.org/10.3389/fpsyg.2018.00798.

21 Sahib S. Khalsa et al., "Interoception and Mental Health: A Roadmap," *Biological Psychiatry: Cognitive Neuroscience and Neuroimaging* 3, no. 6 (June 2018): 501–13, doi.org/10.1016/j.bpsc.2017.12.004.

22 Price and Hooven, "Interoceptive Awareness Skills."

23 Peter Payne, Peter A. Levine, and Mardi A. Crane-Godreau, "Somatic Experiencing: Using Interoception and Proprioception as Core Elements of Trauma Therapy," *Frontiers in Psychology* 6 (2015): 93, doi.org/10.3389/fpsyg.2015.00093.

24 Kuhfuß et al., "Somatic Experiencing."

25 Jonathan Gibson, "Mindfulness, Interoception, and the Body: A Contemporary Perspective," *Frontiers in Psychology* 10 (2019): 2012, frontiersin.org/article/10.3389/fpsyg.2019.02012.

26 Lisa Feldman Barrett, "The Theory of Constructed Emotion: An Active Inference Account of Interoception and Categorization," *Social Cognitive and Affective Neuroscience* 12, no. 1 (January 2017): 1–23, doi.org/10.1093/scan/nsw154.

27 Lisa Feldman Barrett, "That Is Not How Your Brain Works," *Nautilus*, March 3, 2021, nautil.us/that-is-not-how-your-brain-works-238138.

28 Lisa Feldman Barrett, *How Emotions Are Made: The Secret Life of the Brain* (New York: Houghton Mifflin Harcourt, 2017), 82–83.

29 Barrett, *How Emotions Are Made*, 77–78.

30 Barrett, *How Emotions Are Made*, 176–77.

31 Price and Hooven, "Interoceptive Awareness Skills."

32 Mallory Feldman and Kristen A. Lindquist, "What Makes a Woman's Body," *Aeon*, January 21, 2021, aeon.co/essays/womens-bodies-emerge-on-the-shoreline-between-biology-and-culture.

33 Lacie L. Parker and Jennifer A. Harriger, "Eating Disorders and Disordered Eating Behaviors in the LGBT Population: A Review of the Literature," *Journal of Eating Disorders* 8, no. 1 (October 16, 2020): 51, doi.org/10.1186/s40337-020-00327-y.

34 Jennifer K. MacCormack and Kristen A. Lindquist, "Bodily Contributions to Emotion: Schachter's Legacy for a Psychological Constructionist View on Emotion," *Emotion Review* 9, no. 1 (2017): 36–45, doi.org/10.1177/1754073916639664.

35 Price and Weng, "Facilitating Adaptive Emotion Processing."

9: There's a Pill for That

1 Glennon Doyle, Abby Wambach, and Amanda Doyle, "Episode 01: Anxiety: Is It Just Love Holding Its Breath?," May 11, 2021, in *We Can Do Hard Things*, produced by Cadence 13, podcast, 62:05, momastery.com/blog/episode-01.

2 Queensland Brain Institute, "What Are Neurotransmitters?," University of Queensland Australia, November 9, 2017, qbi.uq.edu.au/brain/brain-physiology/what-are-neurotransmitters.

3 Organisation for Economic Co-operation and Development, *Health at a Glance 2017: OECD Indicators* (Paris: OECD Publishing, 2017), 190, doi.org/10.1787/health_glance-2017-en.

4 Ellen Van Leeuwen et al., "Approaches for Discontinuation Versus Continuation of Long-Term Antidepressant Use for Depressive and Anxiety Disorders in Adults," *Cochrane Database of Systematic Reviews* 4 (April 22, 2021): CD013495, doi.org/10.1002/14651858.CD013495.pub2.

5 Debra J. Brody and Qiuping Gu, "Antidepressant Use Among Adults: United States, 2015–2018," NCHS Data Brief, No. 377 (Hyattsville, MD: Centers for Disease Control and Prevention, 2020), cdc.gov/nchs/products/databriefs/db377.htm.

6 Australian Institute of Health and Welfare, "Mental Health–Related Prescriptions," Australian Government, accessed June 29, 2023, aihw.gov.au/mental-health/topic-areas/mental-health-prescriptions.

7 Brody and Gu, "Antidepressant Use Among Adults."

8 Michael Moore et al., "Explaining the Rise in Antidepressant Prescribing: A Descriptive Study Using the General Practice Research Database," *BMJ* 339 (October 15, 2009): b3999, doi.org/10.1136/bmj.b3999.

9 Cochrane Australia, "Antidepressant Use in Australia: A Snapshot," Cochrane Australia, August 27, 2021, australia.cochrane.org/sites/australia.cochrane.org/files/public/uploads/cochrane_antidepressants_discontinuation_review_2021_-_infographic.pdf.

10 Andrea Cipriani et al., "Comparative Efficacy and Acceptability of 21 Antidepressant Drugs for the Acute Treatment of Adults With Major Depressive Disorder: A Systematic Review and Network Meta-Analysis," *The Lancet* 391, no. 10128 (April 7, 2018): 1357–66, doi.org/10.1016/S0140-6736(17)32802-7.

11 Sarah Boseley, "The Drugs Do Work: Antidepressants Are Effective, Study Shows," *The Guardian*, February 21, 2018, theguardian.com/science/2018/feb/21/the-drugs-do-work-antidepressants-are-effective-study-shows.

12 Tarang Sharma et al., "Drop-Out Rates in Placebo-Controlled Trials of Antidepressant Drugs: A Systematic Review and Meta-Analysis Based on Clinical Study Reports," *International Journal of Risk & Safety in Medicine* 30, no. 4 (2019): 217–32, doi.org/10.3233/JRS-195041.

13 Royal College of Psychiatrists, "PS04/19: Position Statement on Antidepressants and Depression" (London: Royal College of Psychiatrists, May 2019), www.rcpsych.ac.uk/docs/default-source/improving-care/better-mh-policy/position-statements/ps04_19---antidepressants-and-depression.pdf.

14 Anne Rochon Ford and Diane Saibil, eds., *The Push to Prescribe: Women and Canadian Drug Policy* (Toronto: Women's Press, 2009), 42.

15 Jonathan M. Metzl, "'Mother's Little Helper': The Crisis of Psychoanalysis and the Miltown Resolution," *Gender & History* 15, no. 2 (2003): 228–55, doi.org/10.1111/1468-0424.00300.

16 Metzl, "'Mother's Little Helper.'"

17 Ellie King, "Sex Bias in Psychoactive Drug Advertisements," *Psychiatry* 43, no. 2 (May 1980): 129–37, doi.org/10.1080/00332747.1980.11024058.

18 Benedict Carey, "Frank Berger, 94, Miltown Creator, Dies," *New York Times*, March 21, 2008, nytimes.com/2008/03/21/health/research/21berger.html.

19 Phillip Curry and Marita O'Brien, "The Male Heart and the Female Mind: A Study in the Gendering of Antidepressants and Cardiovascular Drugs in Advertisements in Irish Medical Publication," *Social Science & Medicine* 62, no. 8 (April 2006): 1970–77, doi.org/10.1016/j.socscimed.2005.08.063.

20 Lisa M. Schwartz and Steven Woloshin, "Medical Marketing in the United States, 1997–2016," *JAMA* 321, no. 1 (January 1, 2019): 80–96, doi.org/10.1001/jama.2018.19320.

21 Marcin Rodzinka, Marie Fallon-Kund, and Claudia Marinetti, *Shedding Light on Transparent Cooperation in Health Care: The Way Forward for Sunshine and Transparency Laws Across Europe* (Brussels: Mental Health Europe, 2019), mhe-sme.org/wp-content/uploads/2019/01/MHE-SHEDDING-LIGHT-REPORT-Final.pdf.

22 Lena Thunander Sundbom et al., "Are Men Under-Treated and Women Over-Treated With Antidepressants? Findings From a Cross-Sectional Survey in Sweden," *BJPsych Bulletin* 41, no. 3 (June 2017): 145–50, doi.org/10.1192/pb.bp.116.054270.

23 Vivane Kovess-Masfety et al., "Are There Gender Differences in Service Use for Mental Disorders Across Countries in the European Union? Results From the EU-World Mental Health Survey," *Journal of Epidemiology & Community Health* 68, no. 7 (July 2014): 649–56, doi.org/10.1136/jech-2013-202962.

24 Thunander Sundbom et al., "Are Men Under-Treated and Women Over-Treated."

25 Siddhartha Mukherjee, "Post-Prozac Nation," *New York Times Magazine,* April 19, 2012, nytimes.com/2012/04/22/magazine/the-science-and-history-of-treating-depression.html.

26 Lauren Slater, *Prozac Diary* (London: Penguin Books, 1999).

27 Todd M. Hillhouse and Joseph H. Porter, "A Brief History of the Development of Antidepressant Drugs: From Monoamines to Glutamate," *Experimental and Clinical Psychopharmacology* 23, no. 1 (February 2015): 1–21, doi.org/10.1037/a0038550.

28 Steven E. Hyman, "Neurotransmitters," *Current Biology* 15, no. 5 (March 8, 2005): R154–58, doi.org/10.1016/j.cub.2005.02.037.

29 David A. Barton et al., "Elevated Brain Serotonin Turnover in Patients With Depression: Effect of Genotype and Therapy," *Archives of General Psychiatry* 65, no. 1 (January 1, 2008): 38–46, doi.org/10.1001/archgenpsychiatry.2007.11.

30 Joanna Moncrieff et al., "The Serotonin Theory of Depression: A Systematic Umbrella Review of the Evidence," *Molecular Psychiatry,* July 20, 2022, 1–14, doi.org/10.1038/s41380-022-01661-0.

31 Jeffrey R. Lacasse and Jonathan Leo, "Antidepressants and the Chemical Imbalance Theory of Depression: A Reflection and Update on the Discourse," *Behavior Therapist* 38, no. 7 (November 2015): 206–13, researchgate.net/publication/284720621_Antidepressants_and_the_Chemical_Imbalance_Theory_of_Depression_A_Reflection_and_Update_on_the_Discourse_with_Responses_from_Ronald_Pies_and_Daniel_Carlat.

32 Y. Zhou and N. C. Danbolt, "Glutamate as a Neurotransmitter in the Healthy Brain," *Journal of Neural Transmission* 121, no. 8 (August 2014): 799–817, doi.org/10.1007/s00702-014-1180-8.

33 Jayashri Kulkarni et al., "Effect of the Glutamate NMDA Receptor Antagonist Memantine as Adjunctive Treatment in Borderline Personality Disorder: An Exploratory, Randomised, Double-Blind, Placebo-Controlled Trial," *CNS Drugs* 32, no. 2 (February 2018): 179–87, doi.org/10.1007/s40263-018-0506-8.

34 Rebecca L. Dean et al., "Ketamine and Other Glutamate Receptor Modulators for Depression in Adults With Bipolar Disorder," *Cochrane Database of Systematic Reviews* 10 (October 8, 2021): CD011611, doi.org/10.1002/14651858.CD011611.pub3.

35 John J. Sramek, Michael F. Murphy, and Neal R. Cutler, "Sex Differences in the Psychopharmacological Treatment of Depression," *Dialogues in Clinical Neuroscience* 18, no. 4 (December 2016): 447–57, doi.org/10.31887/DCNS.2016.18.4/ncutler.

36 Paul Andrews and Jay Amsterdam, "A Hormetic Approach to Understanding Antidepressant Effectiveness and the Development of Antidepressant

Tolerance—a Conceptual View," *Psychiatria Polska* 54, no. 6 (June 2020): 1067–90, doi.org/10.12740/PP/120084.

37   Julie M. Green, "What I Wish I'd Known Before Tapering Off My Antidepressant," *Chatelaine*, September 20, 2021, chatelaine.com/health/antidepressant-withdrawal.

38   Sramek, Murphy, and Cutler, "Sex Differences."

39   Irving Zucker and Brian J. Prendergast, "Sex Differences in Pharmacokinetics Predict Adverse Drug Reactions in Women," *Biology of Sex Differences* 11, no. 1 (June 2020): 32, doi.org/10.1186/s13293-020-00308-5.

40   Philippe Kerr et al., "Allostatic Load and Women's Brain Health: A Systematic Review," *Frontiers in Neuroendocrinology* 59 (October 2020): 100858, doi.org/10.1016/j.yfrne.2020.100858.

41   Caroline Criado Perez, *Invisible Women: Data Bias in a World Designed for Men* (New York: Abrams Press, 2019), 204.

42   Zucker and Prendergast, "Sex Differences in Pharmacokinetics."

43   Claire Cartwright et al., "Long-Term Antidepressant Use: Patient Perspectives of Benefits and Adverse Effects," *Patient Preference and Adherence* 10 (July 28, 2016): 1401–7, doi.org/10.2147/PPA.S110632.

44   Alexis J. Bick et al., "Pharmacokinetics, Metabolism and Serum Concentrations of Progestins Used in Contraception," *Pharmacology & Therapeutics* 222 (June 2021): 107789, doi.org/10.1016/j.pharmthera.2020.107789.

45   Anne Guy et al., "The 'Patient Voice': Patients Who Experience Antidepressant Withdrawal Symptoms Are Often Dismissed, or Misdiagnosed With Relapse, or a New Medical Condition," *Therapeutic Advances in Psychopharmacology* 10 (2020): 2045125320967183, doi.org/10.1177/2045125320967183.

46   Paula A. Rochon et al., "Polypharmacy, Inappropriate Prescribing, and Deprescribing in Older People: Through a Sex and Gender Lens," *The Lancet Healthy Longevity* 2, no. 5 (May 1, 2021): e290–300, doi.org/10.1016/S2666-7568(21)00054-4.

47   Lisa M. McCarthy et al., "ThinkCascades: A Tool for Identifying Clinically Important Prescribing Cascades Affecting Older People," *Drugs & Aging* 39, no. 10 (October 2022): 829–40, doi.org/10.1007/s40266-022-00964-9.

48   Maureen McHugh and Joan C. Chrisler, eds., *The Wrong Prescription for Women: How Medicine and Media Create a "Need" for Treatments, Drugs and Surgery* (Santa Barbara, CA: ABC-CLIO, 2015), 240.

49   Lauren Slater, *Blue Dreams: The Science and the Story of the Drugs That Changed Our Minds* (New York: Little Brown and Company, 2018), x.

50   David Goldbloom, *We Can Do Better: Urgent Innovations to Improve Mental Health Access and Care* (New York: Simon and Schuster, 2021), 117.

51   Alessandro Serretti, "The Present and Future of Precision Medicine in Psychiatry: Focus on Clinical Psychopharmacology of Antidepressants," *Clinical Psychopharmacology and Neuroscience* 16, no. 1 (February 2018): 1–6, doi.org/10.9758/cpn.2018.16.1.1.

52   Raffaella Zanardi et al., "Precision Psychiatry in Clinical Practice,"
     International Journal of Psychiatry in Clinical Practice 25, no. 1 (March 2021):
     19–27, doi.org/10.1080/13651501.2020.1809680.

53   Joshua D. Rosenblat, Yena Lee, and Roger S. McIntyre, "Does
     Pharmacogenomic Testing Improve Clinical Outcomes for Major Depressive
     Disorder? A Systematic Review of Clinical Trials and Cost-Effectiveness
     Studies," *Journal of Clinical Psychiatry* 78, no. 6 (June 2017): 720–29, doi.
     org/10.4088/JCP.15r10583; Nazia Darvesh, Jennifer Horton, and Mê-Linh Lê,
     "Pharmacogenomic Testing in Depression: A 2021 Update," *Canadian Journal of
     Health Technologies* 2, no. 1 (January 2022), doi.org/10.51731/cjht.2022.241.

54   Ontario Health (Quality), "Multi-Gene Pharmacogenomic Testing That
     Includes Decision-Support Tools to Guide Medication Selection for Major
     Depression: A Health Technology Assessment," *Ontario Health Technology
     Assessment Series* 21, no. 13 (August 2021): 1–214.

55   Manish K. Jha et al., "Can C-Reactive Protein Inform Antidepressant
     Medication Selection in Depressed Outpatients? Findings From the CO-MED
     Trial," *Psychoneuroendocrinology* 78 (April 2017): 105–13, doi.org/10.1016/j.
     psyneuen.2017.01.023.

56   Madhukar H. Trivedi, "Establishing Moderators and Biosignatures of
     Antidepressant Response for Clinical Care (EMBARC) for Depression," Clinical
     Trial Registration, U.S. National Library of Medicine, December 3, 2018,
     clinicaltrials.gov/ct2/show/NCT01407094.

57   Madhukar H. Trivedi et al., "Establishing Moderators and Biosignatures
     of Antidepressant Response in Clinical Care (EMBARC): Rationale and
     Design," *Journal of Psychiatric Research* 78 (July 2016): 11–23, doi.org/10.1016/j.
     jpsychires.2016.03.001.

10: Making Peace With Our Moods

1   *The Complete Journals of L. M. Montgomery: The PEI Years, 1901–1911*, eds. Mary
    Henley Rubio and Elizabeth Hillman Waterston (Oxford: Oxford University
    Press, 2013), 282.

2   Alanna Mitchell, "Lucy Maud Montgomery's Agonizing Drug Addiction,"
    Maclean's, February 12, 2020, macleans.ca/society/health/lucy-maud-
    montgomerys-secret-drug-addiction.

3   Michael Bauer et al., "World Federation of Societies of Biological Psychiatry
    (WFSBP) Guidelines for Biological Treatment of Unipolar Depressive Disorders.
    Part 2: Maintenance Treatment of Major Depressive Disorder—Update 2015,"
    World Journal of Biological Psychiatry 16, no. 2 (February 2015): 76–95, doi.org/
    10.3109/15622975.2014.1001786.

4   Emma Maund et al., "Managing Antidepressant Discontinuation: A Systematic
    Review," *Annals of Family Medicine* 17, no. 1 (January 2019): 52–60,
    doi.org/10.1370/afm.2336.

5 Ellen Piek, Klaas van der Meer, and Willem A. Nolen, "Guideline Recommend-ations for Long-Term Treatment of Depression With Antidepressants in Primary Care—a Critical Review," *European Journal of General Practice* 16, no. 2 (June 2010): 106–12, doi.org/10.3109/13814781003692463; World Health Organization, "Duration of Antidepressant Treatment," World Health Organization, 2012, who.int/teams/mental-health-and-substance-use/treatment-care/mental-health-gap-action-programme/evidence-centre/depression/duration-of-antidepressant-treatment.

6 Royal College of Psychiatrists, "PS04/19: Position Statement on Antidepressants and Depression," May 2019, www.rcpsych.ac.uk/docs/default-source/improving-care/better-mh-policy/position-statements/ps04_19---antidepressants-and-depression.pdf.

7 National Institute for Health and Care Excellence, *Depression in Adults: Treatment and Management*, NICE Guideline, June 29, 2022, nice.org.uk/guidance/ng222/resources/depression-in-adults-treatment-and-management-pdf-66143832307909.

8 Maund et al., "Managing Antidepressant Discontinuation."

9 Claire Cartwright et al., "Long-Term Antidepressant Use: Patient Perspectives of Benefits and Adverse Effects," *Patient Preference and Adherence* 10 (2016): 1401–7, doi.org/10.2147/PPA.S110632.

10 James Davies and John Read, "A Systematic Review Into the Incidence, Severity and Duration of Antidepressant Withdrawal Effects: Are Guidelines Evidence-Based?," *Addictive Behaviors* 97 (October 2019): 111–21, doi.org/10.1016/j.addbeh.2018.08.027.

11 Anne Guy et al., "The 'Patient Voice': Patients Who Experience Antidepressant Withdrawal Symptoms Are Often Dismissed, or Misdiagnosed With Relapse, or a New Medical Condition," *Therapeutic Advances in Psychopharmacology* 10 (2020): 2045125320967183, doi.org/10.1177/2045125320967183.

12 Southampton Clinical Trials Unit, "REDUCE," University of Southampton, accessed December 9, 2021, southampton.ac.uk/ctu/trialportfolio/lighttouchtrials/reduce.page.

13 Benedict Carey and Robert Gebeloff, "Many People Taking Antidepressants Discover They Cannot Quit," *New York Times*, April 7, 2018, nytimes.com/2018/04/07/health/antidepressants-withdrawal-prozac-cymbalta.html.

14 Brooke Siem, *May Cause Side Effects: A Memoir* (Las Vegas: Central Recovery Press, 2022).

15 Edward White, John Read, and Sherry Julo, "The Role of Facebook Groups in the Management and Raising of Awareness of Antidepressant Withdrawal: Is Social Media Filling the Void Left by Health Services?," *Therapeutic Advances in Psychopharmacology* 11 (2021): 2045125320981174, doi.org/10.1177/2045125320981174.

16 White, Read, and Julo, "The Role of Facebook Groups."

17 Karen L. Fortuna et al., "Digital Peer Support Mental Health Interventions for People With a Lived Experience of a Serious Mental Illness: Systematic Review," *JMIR Mental Health* 7, no. 4 (April 3, 2020): e16460, doi.org/10.2196/16460.

18 Guy et al., "The 'Patient Voice.'"

19 Emma Maund et al., "Barriers and Facilitators to Discontinuing Antidepressant Use: A Systematic Review and Thematic Synthesis," *Journal of Affective Disorders* 245 (February 15, 2019): 38–62, doi.org/10.1016/j.jad.2018.10.107.

20 Phillippa Harrison et al., "Study Protocol for the Antidepressant Advisor (ADESS): A Decision Support System for Antidepressant Treatment for Depression in UK Primary Care: A Feasibility Study," *BMJ Open* 10, no. 5 (May 1, 2020): e035905, doi.org/10.1136/bmjopen-2019-035905.

21 Paul W. Andrews and J. Anderson Thomson, "Depression's Evolutionary Roots," *Scientific American*, August 25, 2009, scientificamerican.com/article/depressions-evolutionary.

22 Kristen L. Syme and Edward H. Hagen, "Mental Health Is Biological Health: Why Tackling 'Diseases of the Mind' Is an Imperative for Biological Anthropology in the 21st Century," *American Journal of Biological Anthropology* 171, no. S70 (May 2020): 87–117, doi.org/10.1002/ajpa.23965.

23 Lisa Feldman Barrett, *How Emotions Are Made: The Secret Life of the Brain* (New York: Houghton Mifflin Harcourt, 2017), 212–14.

24 Daniel P. Johnson and Mark A. Whisman, "Gender Differences in Rumination: A Meta-Analysis," *Personality and Individual Differences* 55, no. 4 (August 2013): 367–74, doi.org/10.1016/j.paid.2013.03.019.

25 Stephanie A. Kolakowsky-Hayner et al., "Psychosocial Impacts of the COVID-19 Quarantine: A Study of Gender Differences in 59 Countries," *Medicina* 57, no. 8 (August 2021): 789, doi.org/10.3390/medicina57080789.

26 Mallory Feldman and Kristen A. Lindquist, "What Makes a Woman's Body," *Aeon*, January 21, 2021, aeon.co/essays/womens-bodies-emerge-on-the-shoreline-between-biology-and-culture.

27 Kate Bowler, *No Cure for Being Human: And Other Truths I Need to Hear* (New York: Random House, 2021).

11: From Hysteria to Healing

1 Richard Rohr, *Everything Belongs: The Gift of Contemplative Prayer* (New York: Crossroad Publishing Company, 2003), 19.

2 Emily Nagoski and Amelia Nagoski, *Burnout: The Secret to Unlocking the Stress Cycle* (New York: Ballantine Books, 2019), 101.

3 Hillary L. McBride, *The Wisdom of Your Body: Finding Healing, Wholeness and Connection Through Embodied Living* (Toronto: Collins, 2021), 12.

4 Philip Mackowiak, "Recycling Metchnikoff: Probiotics, the Intestinal Microbiome and the Quest for Long Life," *Frontiers in Public Health* 1 (November 2013): 52, doi.org/10.3389/fpubh.2013.00052.

5 Alex Riley, *A Cure for Darkness: The Story of Depression and How We Treat It* (New York: Scribner, 2021), 312–13.

6 Richard T. Liu, Rachel F. L. Walsh, and Ana E. Sheehan, "Prebiotics and Probiotics for Depression and Anxiety: A Systematic Review and Meta-Analysis of Controlled Clinical Trials," *Neuroscience & Biobehavioral Reviews* 102 (July 2019): 13–23, doi.org/10.1016/j.neubiorev.2019.03.023.

7 Sigrid Breit et al., "Vagus Nerve as Modulator of the Brain–Gut Axis in Psychiatric and Inflammatory Disorders," *Frontiers in Psychiatry* 9 (March 2018): 44, frontiersin.org/article/10.3389/fpsyt.2018.00044.

8 Narek Israelyan et al., "Effects of Serotonin and Slow-Release 5-Hydroxytryptophan on Gastrointestinal Motility in a Mouse Model of Depression," *Gastroenterology* 157, no. 2 (August 2019): 507–21, e4, doi.org/10.1053/j.gastro.2019.04.022.

9 Anahad O'Connor, "Should You Get a Microbiome Test?," *New York Times*, October 13, 2021, nytimes.com/2021/10/13/well/live/microbiome-test.html.

10 Viome, "Full Body Intelligence™ Test," Viome, accessed December 10, 2022, viome.com/products/full-body-intelligence.

11 Caroline J. K. Wallace and Roumen V. Milev, "The Efficacy, Safety, and Tolerability of Probiotics on Depression: Clinical Results From an Open-Label Pilot Study," *Frontiers in Psychiatry* 12 (February 2021): 618279, doi.org/10.3389/fpsyt.2021.618279; Kenji Sanada et al., "Gut Microbiota and Major Depressive Disorder: A Systematic Review and Meta-Analysis," *Journal of Affective Disorders* 266 (April 1, 2020): 1–13, doi.org/10.1016/j.jad.2020.01.102.

12 Jon Kabat-Zinn, "Too Early to Tell: The Potential Impact and Challenges—Ethical and Otherwise—Inherent in the Mainstreaming of Dharma in an Increasingly Dystopian World," *Mindfulness* 8, no. 5 (October 2017): 1125–35, doi.org/10.1007/s12671-017-0758-2.

13 Royce William Knight et al., "Cost-Effectiveness of the Mindfulness-Based Stress Reduction Methodology," *Mindfulness* 6, no. 6 (December 2015): 1379–86, doi.org/10.1007/s12671-015-0408-5.

14 Anuradha Baminiwatta and Indrajith Solangaarachchi, "Trends and Developments in Mindfulness Research Over 55 Years: A Bibliometric Analysis of Publications Indexed in Web of Science," *Mindfulness* 12, no. 9 (September 2021): 2099–116, doi.org/10.1007/s12671-021-01681-x.

15 Victoria Follette, Kathleen M. Palm, and Adria N. Pearson, "Mindfulness and Trauma: Implications for Treatment," *Journal of Rational-Emotive & Cognitive-Behavior Therapy* 24, no. 1 (March 2006): 45–61, doi.org/10.1007/s10942-006-0025-2.

16 Elizabeth A. Hoge et al., "Mindfulness-Based Stress Reduction vs Escitalopram for the Treatment of Adults With Anxiety Disorders: A Randomized Clinical Trial," *JAMA Psychiatry* 80, no. 1 (January 2023): 13–21, doi.org/10.1001/jamapsychiatry.2022.3679.

17 Chris C. Streeter et al., "Effects of Yoga Versus Walking on Mood, Anxiety, and Brain GABA Levels: A Randomized Controlled MRS Study," *Journal of Alternative and Complementary Medicine* 16, no. 11 (November 2010): 1145–52, doi.org/10.1089/acm.2010.0007.

18   Shivarama Varambally, Sanju George, and Bangalore Nanjundaiah Gangadhar, "Yoga for Psychiatric Disorders: From Fad to Evidence-Based Intervention?," *British Journal of Psychiatry* 216, no. 6 (June 2020): 291–93, doi.org/10.1192/bjp.2019.249.

19   Patricia Cabral, Hilary B. Meyer, and Donna Ames, "Effectiveness of Yoga Therapy as a Complementary Treatment for Major Psychiatric Disorders: A Meta-Analysis," *Primary Care Companion for CNS Disorders* 13, no. 4 (2011): PCC.10r01068, doi.org/10.4088/PCC.10r01068.

20   Canadian Agency for Drugs and Technologies in Health, "Yoga for the Treatment of Post-Traumatic Stress Disorder, Generalized Anxiety Disorder, Depression, and Substance Abuse: A Review of the Clinical Effectiveness and Guidelines," CADTH Rapid Response Service, June 22, 2015, 46, cadth.ca/sites/default/files/pdf/htis/june-2015/RC0670_Yoga_Final.pdf.

21   Ankita Rao, "To Some, Mindfulness Feels Too Whitewashed to Embrace," *Vice*, June 29, 2018, vice.com/en/article/mbkzdq/mindfulness-apps-whitewashed-spirituality.

22   Caoimhe Twohig-Bennett and Andy Jones, "The Health Benefits of the Great Outdoors: A Systematic Review and Meta-Analysis of Greenspace Exposure and Health Outcomes," *Environmental Research* 166 (October 2018): 628–37, doi.org/10.1016/j.envres.2018.06.030.

23   Joseph Cipriani et al., "A Systematic Review of the Effects of Horticultural Therapy on Persons With Mental Health Conditions," *Occupational Therapy in Mental Health* 33, no. 1 (January 2, 2017): 47–69, doi.org/10.1080/0164212X.2016.1231602.

24   Daniel J. Bowen, James T. Neill, and Simon J. R. Crisp, "Wilderness Adventure Therapy Effects on the Mental Health of Youth Participants," *Evaluation and Program Planning* 58 (October 2016): 49–59, doi.org/10.1016/j.evalprogplan.2016.05.005.

25   MaryCarol R. Hunter, Brenda W. Gillespie, and Sophie Yu-Pu Chen, "Urban Nature Experiences Reduce Stress in the Context of Daily Life Based on Salivary Biomarkers," *Frontiers in Psychology* 10 (April 2019): 722, doi.org/10.3389/fpsyg.2019.00722.

26   Dorthe Djernis et al., "A Systematic Review and Meta-Analysis of Nature-Based Mindfulness: Effects of Moving Mindfulness Training Into an Outdoor Natural Setting," *International Journal of Environmental Research and Public Health* 16, no. 17 (September 2019): 3202, doi.org/10.3390/ijerph16173202.

27   David H. Rosmarin, Kenneth I. Pargament, and Harold G. Koenig, "Spirituality and Mental Health: Challenges and Opportunities," *The Lancet Psychiatry* 8, no. 2 (February 2021): 92–93, doi.org/10.1016/S2215-0366(20)30048-1.

28   Rosmarin, Pargament, and Koenig, "Spirituality and Mental Health."

29   Gregory A. Smith, "About Three-in-Ten U.S. Adults Are Now Religiously Unaffiliated," Pew Research Center's Religion and Public Life Project (blog), December 14, 2021, pewforum.org/2021/12/14/about-three-in-ten-u-s-adults-are-now-religiously-unaffiliated.

30 Pew Research Center, "Being Christian in Western Europe," Pew Research Center's Religion and Public Life Project (blog), May 29, 2018, pewforum. org/2018/05/29/being-christian-in-western-europe.

31 Harriet Sherwood, "Religion: Why Faith Is Becoming More and More Popular," *The Guardian*, August 27, 2018, theguardian.com/news/2018/aug/27/ religion-why-is-faith-growing-and-what-happens-next.

32 Michael Lipka and Claire Gecewicz, "More Americans Now Say They're Spiritual but Not Religious," Pew Research Center, September 6, 2017, pewresearch.org/short-reads/2017/09/06/more-americans-now-say-theyre-spiritual-but-not-religious.

33 David Saunders et al., "Varieties of Religious (Non)Affiliation: A Primer for Mental Health Practitioners on the 'Spiritual but Not Religious' and the 'Nones,'" *Journal of Nervous and Mental Disease* 208, no. 5 (May 2020): 424–30, doi.org/10.1097/NMD.0000000000001141.

34 Michael King et al., "Religion, Spirituality and Mental Health: Results From a National Study of English Households," *British Journal of Psychiatry* 202, no. 1 (January 2013): 68–73, doi.org/10.1192/bjp.bp.112.112003.

35 Harold G. Koenig, "Research on Religion, Spirituality, and Mental Health: A Review," *Canadian Journal of Psychiatry* 54, no. 5 (May 2009): 283–91, doi.org/10.1177/070674370905400502.

36 John M. Salsman et al., "A Meta-Analytic Approach to Examining the Correlation Between Religion/Spirituality and Mental Health in Cancer," *Cancer* 121, no. 21 (November 1, 2015): 3769–78, doi.org/10.1002/cncr.29350.

37 Andrew Newberg, "Mind and God: The New Science of Neurotheology," *Big Think*, May 6, 2021, bigthink.com/neuropsych/mind-god-new-science-neurotheology.

38 Nancy A. Wintering et al., "Effect of a One-Week Spiritual Retreat on Brain Functional Connectivity: A Preliminary Study," *Religions* 12, no. 1 (January 2021): 23, doi.org/10.3390/rel12010023.

39 Timothy B. Smith, Jeremy Bartz, and P. Scott Richards, "Outcomes of Religious and Spiritual Adaptations to Psychotherapy: A Meta-Analytic Review," *Psychotherapy Research* 17, no. 6 (October 2007): 643–55, doi.org/10.1080/10503300701250347.

40 David H. Rosmarin et al., "Predictors of Patients' Responses to Spiritual Psychotherapy for Inpatient, Residential, and Intensive Treatment (SPIRIT)," *Psychiatric Services* 72, no. 5 (May 2021): 507–13, doi.org/10.1176/appi. ps.202000331; J. P. B. Gonçalves et al., "Religious and Spiritual Interventions in Mental Health Care: A Systematic Review and Meta-Analysis of Randomized Controlled Clinical Trials," *Psychological Medicine* 45, no. 14 (October 2015): 2937–49, doi.org/10.1017/S0033291715001166.

41 Jolyn Sloan, "'Unravelling': Exploring the Experience and Meaning of Spiritual Deconstruction" (master's thesis, University of Saskatchewan, 2021), harvest. usask.ca/bitstream/handle/10388/13602/SLOAN-THESIS-2021.pdf.

42 Deborah Farmer Kris, "Awe Might Be Our Most Undervalued Emotion. Here's

How to Help Children Find It," *Washington Post*, November 30, 2021, washingtonpost.com/lifestyle/on-parenting/children-awe-emotion/2021/11/29/0f78a4b0-4c8e-11ec-b0b0-766bbbe79347_story.html.

43 Jennifer E. Stellar et al., "Positive Affect and Markers of Inflammation: Discrete Positive Emotions Predict Lower Levels of Inflammatory Cytokines," *Emotion* 15, no. 2 (April 2015): 129–33, doi.org/10.1037/emo0000033.

44 Craig L. Anderson, Maria Monroy, and Dacher Keltner, "Awe in Nature Heals: Evidence From Military Veterans, At-Risk Youth, and College Students," *Emotion* 18, no. 8 (December 2018): 1195–1202, doi.org/10.1037/emo0000442.

45 Ethan Kross, *Chatter: The Voice in Our Head, Why It Matters, and How to Harness It* (New York: Crown, 2021), 121–22.

46 Jeanne Nakamura and Mihaly Csikszentmihalyi, "The Concept of Flow," in *Flow and the Foundations of Positive Psychology: The Collected Works of Mihaly Csikszentmihalyi*, ed. Mihaly Csikszentmihalyi (Dordrecht: Springer Netherlands, 2014), 239–63, doi.org/10.1007/978-94-017-9088-8_16.

47 Eve Rodsky, *Find Your Unicorn Space: Reclaim Your Creative Life in a Too-Busy World* (New York: G.P. Putnam's Sons, 2021), 74.

48 Yang Bai et al., "Awe, the Diminished Self, and Collective Engagement: Universals and Cultural Variations in the Small Self," *Journal of Personality and Social Psychology* 113, no. 2 (August 2017): 185–209, doi.org/10.1037/pspa0000087.

49 Nakamura and Csikszentmihalyi, "The Concept of Flow."

50 Tamlin S. Conner, Colin G. DeYoung, and Paul J. Silvia, "Everyday Creative Activity as a Path to Flourishing," *Journal of Positive Psychology* 13, no. 2 (March 4, 2018): 181–89, doi.org/10.1080/17439760.2016.1257049.

51 Rodsky, *Find Your Unicorn Space*, 136.

52 Nuria Codina and José V. Pestana, "Time Matters Differently in Leisure Experience for Men and Women: Leisure Dedication and Time Perspective," *International Journal of Environmental Research and Public Health* 16, no. 14 (July 14, 2019): E2513, doi.org/10.3390/ijerph16142513.

53 Wendy Wang, "The 'Leisure Gap' Between Mothers and Fathers," Pew Research Center, October 17, 2013, pewresearch.org/fact-tank/2013/10/17/the-leisure-gap-between-mothers-and-fathers; Esteban Ortiz-Ospina, Charlie Giattino, and Max Roser, "Time Use," Our World in Data, November 29, 2020, ourworldindata.org/time-use.

Epilogue

1 CBC Radio, "Tapestry at 25: Irish Poet John O'Donohue," October 4, 2019, cbc.ca/radio/tapestry/tapestry-at-25-john-o-donohue-and-mavis-staples-1.5309014/tapestry-at-25-irish-poet-john-o-donohue-1.5309033.

2 Juliet Young (@Juliet_Young1), "An update on a previous drawing," Twitter, February 18, 2022, 1:36 p.m., twitter.com/Juliet_Young1/status/1494742723500331009.

INDEX

Figures indicated by page numbers in italics